SHAOLIN NEI JIN QI GONG

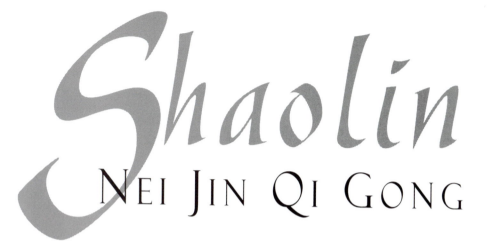

Shaolin
NEI JIN QI GONG

Ancient Healing
in the Modern World

PETER FENTON, Ph.D.

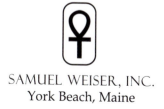

SAMUEL WEISER, INC.
York Beach, Maine

First published in the United States in 1996 by
SAMUEL WEISER, INC.
P.O. Box 612
York Beach, ME 03910-0612

Library of Congress Cataloging-in-Publication Data

Fenton, Peter.
   Shaolin Nei Jing Qi Gong : ancient healing in the
modern world / Peter Fenton.
      p. cm.
   Includes bibliographical references.
   1. Ch'i kung. I. Title.
RA781.8.F467   1996
613.7'1--dc20   96-15198
                                                      CIP

ISBN 0-87728-876-3
MG

Cover photography by Jim Ford.
Photographs in text by Jim Ford.
Illustrations by Jean Herzel.

Typeset in 10.5 Book Antiqua
Cover and text design by Kathryn Sky-Peck

Printed in the United States of America

02 01 00
10 9 8 7 6 5 4 3 2

The paper used in this publication meets or exceeds the minimum requirements
of the American National Standard for Permanence of Paper of Printed Library
Materials Z39.48-1984.

FOR GRAND MASTER PENG JIU LING, who brought these teachings to the West and to the students of his school, past, present, and future.

CONTENTS

CHAPTER 1: BACKGROUND, 1

CHAPTER 2: THE DISCIPLINE, 29

CHAPTER 3: THE HEALING ASPECTS OF
QI AND QI GONG, 97

CHAPTER 4: MEDITATIONS, 117

CHAPTER 5: THE CHANNELS, 127

LIST OF DIAGRAMS, PHOTOS AND ILLUSTRATIONS

CHAPTER 1: BACKGROUND

CHAPTER 2: THE DISCIPLINE

Warm Up Exercises

Circle the Shoulder

Series 1

Horse Stance

Finger Bending

Embracing the Moon with Both Hands

Series 2

Series 3

Series 4

Closing Exercise

CHAPTER 3: THE HEALING ASPECTS OF QI AND QI GONG METHODOLOGY

CHAPTER 4: MEDITATIONS

CHAPTER 5: THE CHANNELS

Publisher's Note

The author and publisher of this material are not responsible in any manner whatsoever for any injury caused directly or indirectly by reading or following the instructions in this text. The physical and psychological activities described in the text may be too strenuous for some people. Readers of this text should consult a qualified physician before engaging in these, or any other, exercises.

If you have a medical condition or are of uncertain health, immediately seek attention and advice from a qualified medical doctor. Although the practice of Qi Gong is beneficial in many instances, it is neither a diagnostic tool nor an exclusive treatment for pathological conditions. Qi Gong can be used to complement, but not to replace, a doctor's care.

Shaolin Nei Jin Qi Gong

CHAPTER 1

Background

In a darkened room in a silent corner of the museum sits a collection of statues, purchased, unearthed, or stolen from a dozen locations in the Far East. Each is displayed in its own case, in its own special section of the room. Some are illuminated with tiny bulbs. Others shine with their own peculiar internal light. All have writeups, cleverly worded, neat and to the point, posted conveniently beneath each pedestal: this work is from Bali, that one from China, the one in the corner from Thailand. The more prominent pieces are accompanied by descriptive pamphlets stored in plastic fixtures. They are written for the mildly curious, and are intended to be read over an expensive cup of coffee in the snack bar, then stuffed in an inside coat pocket or a purse; as much an exercise in public relations as a meaningful document.

But standing in the presence of these wonders from antiquity, all of the trappings, the expensive stands, the decor of the room, even the building itself, fades away into obscurity. Each of the statues here represents a Buddha or a deity. Several—notably the Tibetan works—depict entire scenes with whole groups of characters engaged in bizarre performances. By abstracting the sculpture from its apparent significance, the spectator is in a position to derive an entirely different and deeper level of meaning.

To the untrained eye, these statues are notable for their beauty, their ferocity, their antiquity or any number of other physical characteristics. Some observers even note the historical significance

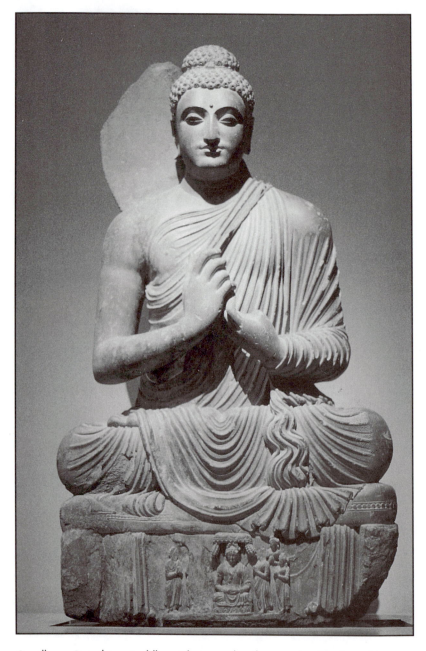

Gandhara Preaching Buddha. (Photograph taken at the Glenbow Museum, Calgary, Alberta, Canada.)

of a piece. Comparatively few, however, recognize that each statue is a repository of esoteric knowledge, bound up in this physical form so that it might withstand the disintegrating influences of time.

The next time you see one of these creations, study its demeanor. Is it fierce or smiling? Is it serene and impassive, or harsh and judgmental? Is it standing or seated? Is it nearly naked, dressed plainly, or covered in fine robes? When you have finished your observations, note the positions of its limbs and, of equal importance, its fingers and palms. These statues, as well as being works of art, are also icons. Their true value is found not in their artistic merit or cultural significance but in the quality of information they transmit. In essence, they are intended to represent a specific aspect of enlightened mind.

The individuals who were (and still are) assigned the duty of preserving a tradition spared no effort to capture specific ideas in their art forms. Details such as the physical architecture, its placement according to the four cardinal directions and the type of hand gesture (mudra) to name but a few qualities, all contribute to the overall strategy of the artists to achieve their goal. In this way, many levels of meaning and function are embodied in the art form.

If you study the mudras, you will discover that these hand gestures serve as a distinct language. Each finger is associated with a particular color, a sound, an element, a heavenly guardian, an organ, and an acupuncture channel. This kind of knowledge helps ensure that the specific meaning conveyed by the statue is not misunderstood. Another purpose served by the language of mudras is to guarantee a means of communication among devotees from diverse language groups. Knowing such a language (there were many, Buddhist ceremonial and Hindu Raja yoga, to name but two) allowed the lama or guru to communicate with students of many diverse nationalities.

A raised right hand, with palm out and thumb tucked in, indicates a gesture of blessing or, more exactly, of instilling fearlessness into the beholder. Other mudras signify postures of meditation, of preaching, of renouncing the world and so on. In the photograph known as the Gandhara Preaching Buddha (after its geographical

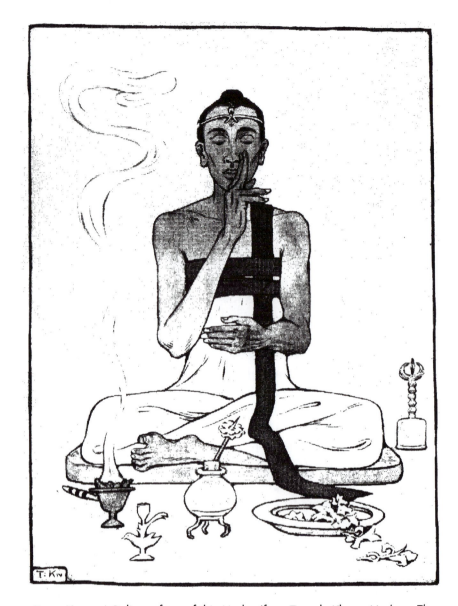

Prana Yama: A Balinese form of this Mudra (from Tyra de Kleen, *Mudras: The Ritual Hand-Poses of the Buddhist Priests and the Shiva Priests of Bali.* London: Kegan Paul, Trench, Turnbull, & Co., Ltd., 1924, page 44).

place of origin in the northern Indus valley), the Buddha is represented as preaching to his congregation (page 2). The position of his hands indicates not only that he is preaching, but also that he is teaching his first sermon. Religious art of this quality, infused as it is with many layers of sacred knowledge, seeks to induce a particular state of mind and being in the beholder. This is one significant difference between religious art and many other art forms.

Another picture, from Tyra de Kleen's book, *Mudras: The Ritual Hand-Poses of the Buddhist Priests and the Shiva Priests of Bali*, illustrates one such mudra (page 4). Describing it she says, "Prana-Yama: (= Breath Control). This Balinese Mudra is called by the same name as the breathing exercise in the Hindu Raja- and the Hatha-yoga system where it plays a very great part in acquiring occult psychic powers. This regulation of the breath is done by closing one nostril with two fingers while evenly and silently drawing in the air through the other; retaining the breath as long as possible; and then closing the other nostril while breathing out through the first." She continues to note that the priest, when displaying this mudra, does not actually do the breathing itself, but only makes the gesture. Interestingly, de Kleen mentions in a footnote to this mudra that Prana does not really mean *breath*, but refers to the *vital energy* (Qi) in the breath, the energy of the universe.[1]

In the larger picture, distinctions in meaning often follow general categories which are reflected in the works of art. This immediately directs the attention along specific lines and has the effect of drawing the spectator into the frame of mind intended by the artist. Generally speaking, it is only the initiates who understand the deeper layers of meaning but, regardless of their degree of involvement with the tradition, many who behold such works immediately sense powerful underlying influences, even to the extent that they stand in awe. Table 1 (page 6) is derived from *The Image of the Buddha*, edited by David L. Snellgrove, and describes several major iconographic distinctions among the five great Buddhic manifestations.

---

1. Tyra de Kleen, *Mudras: The Ritual Hand-Poses of the Buddhist Priests and the Shiva Priests of Bali* (London: Kegan Paul, Trench, Turnbull & Co., Ltd., 1924), pp. 38, 39.

Table 1: Distinctions among the Five Principal Buddhic Manifestations.

Sanskrit Name	English Translation	Cosmic Direction	Mudra (Gesture)
Vairocana	Resplendent	Center	Preaching
Aksobhya	Imperturbable	East	Touching the Earth
Ratnasambhave	Jewel-Born	South	Generosity
Amitabha	Boundless Light	West	Meditation
Amoghasiddhi	Infallible Success	North	Fearlessness

These statues, then, as well as being works of art, are also structured methods for transmitting specific information. Behind each work is a history and in some cases, a set of instructions. This information is carefully compiled, through trial and error techniques, after years or even generations of study and practice. The results of this painstaking work are then carefully recorded in the art form. It should be remembered, though, that these works merely suggest an aspect of the truth understood by the artist. In the final analysis they are no more than a means to an end, and may even hinder the aspirant from achievement. The vast number of religious art forms in certain cultures suggests that their creation has become something of a fixation, perhaps even supplanting in importance the pursuit of esoteric knowledge of greater worth.

Some of these works were concealed in the inner recesses of monasteries. Others became the centerpieces for large public temples. With practice, you may develop your inner senses to the point where you are able to distinguish which of the statues have been heavily worshipped and which have remained veiled. You will be in a better position to explain how this quality of knowledge might be possible after you begin your practice.

As you advance in your Qi Gong discipline, you will begin to realize that the key to deciphering these ancient codes is embedded in these postures, hand and finger gestures. You will understand relationships between stances, internal organs, and groups of organs, between finger positions and channels. You will recognize that both the postures and finger positions strengthen and promote the flow of Qi, the living and universal energy found throughout creation. Most importantly, your understanding will not be restricted to an intellectual knowledge but will be based in the physiology itself. You will feel the Qi of nature from the sands and waters, from the trees and plants. Over time, you will be able to direct its movement within yourself or guide its flow to another for healing purposes.

The version of Qi Gong to be treated in this text is known as Shaolin (after the temple of its origin) Nei (internal) Jin (force) Qi (vital energy) Gong (achievements of practice) and was introduced to the West by Grand Master Peng Jiu Ling, formerly from mainland China. The Shaolin temple is probably the most famous of all Chinese monasteries, and from it come many versions of Qi Gong. Not all styles, however, find their origins in the temple. In fact, the practice of Qi Gong is widespread in Asia and there seem to be almost as many styles, 3,000 or more, as there are individual Masters. Each Master, Grand Master, or Great Grand Master holds a single piece of the Qi Gong puzzle and no one understands the discipline in its entirety. The problem is further compounded when you consider that many forms of Qi Gong are still developing.

Following the guidelines in this text will allow practitioners to accomplish a number of fundamental goals. Because each goal is critical to the practice, all are presented in point form below. After diligent study of this text, students will:

- Understand the concepts of Qi and Qi Gong;
- Understand the relationship between Qi and Traditional Chinese Medicine, particularly the notions of channels and acupuncture;
- Develop a robust practice and establish a reliable foundation for future study;
- Strengthen vital physical energies in the body as a result of practice;

- Be able to use Qi to treat self and others;
- Through the study of this art, the great spirit of Shaolin Nei Jin Qi Gong will be advanced.

QI GONG IN ACTION

Through a translator, the Master from Shanghai asked the client to stand before him, relaxing as much as possible. He then began a Qi massage, rubbing her shoulders, neck, and back with a gentle, circular motion. In a few minutes, the woman's body posture had changed. Moments before, she had been tense, essentially a rigid collection of muscles and bones dominated by the forces of the world around her. She was now only semiconscious, her head bowed so that it almost touched her chest.

At this point, the Master moved to a position ten feet in front of her. Sitting on a small pillow, he assumed a full lotus position. The woman had not moved, still looking more like a wooden puppet than a human being. From my vantage point at the side of the room, I could see the Master nearly close his eyes and then raise his right arm, half bent at the elbow. Pointing his fingers at the motionless woman, he began to push and pull with his arms seemingly at the air before him. Soon, in exact rhythm with these motions, the woman's body began to rock, first back onto the heels of her feet and then onto her toes. This was peculiar, because her eyes were closed and I could not help but speculate as to how this happened. It was a curious sight. How could her body do this and not fall over? Even more inexplicable was the fact that the patient, or at least her body, somehow knew how to keep time with the motion of the Master's hands even though she seemed to be unconscious, with eyes closed.

As she rocked back and forth, I noticed how stiff her body appeared, still rigid, even though it was moving in a definite rhythm. Just the sight of this affected posture gave me a profound insight into the nature of this woman's illness. Without a doubt, I knew that her psychological relationship with her body had somehow been arrested. I also knew that for her to fully recover, she would have to take responsibility for restoring that relationship.

For the moment, though, the Master was reinforcing her life force, her Qi, with that of his own. As well, he was attempting to encourage the movement of Qi in her body pathways that had been long dormant.

Unlike our practice, Shaolin Nei Jin Qi Gong, with this particular Gong, the practitioner transmits personal Qi, life energy stored within the body itself, to another for the purposes of healing. The whole process can be extremely demanding, and even dangerous, to the health. Some Masters have reportedly died from overexertion. As a result, many practitioners of this style will never use their Qi for healing purposes unless a close family member or friend is involved. Even those who do practice healing often hold a deep aversion to it, since using this technique involves an expenditure of personal vitality.

After twenty minutes, the Master stopped, stood up, and once again began to rub his patient's neck, shoulders, and back with the palm of his hand. Using one hand to stabilize her body, he used the other to rub the Qi right through her clothing into the body tissues. His hand moved in circles, first in one direction and then in the other. After a time, he switched hands. At this point, the woman slowly opened her eyes as she recovered consciousness. It reminded me of someone awakening from a deep hypnotic trance. She did not remember what had happened, and only said that she felt well rested and strengthened.

PROPERTIES OF QI

The Qi of nature creates and nourishes everything in the world. It is an intelligent force which exists in us, around us, and throughout the universe. Qi manifests in many ways. When it is inside the human body, it assumes several forms. Its primary characteristic is that it is a vital energy more primordial than blood itself. At birth, it is a force which is transmitted directly from mother to child. This type of Qi is referred to as prenatal Qi. It is intimately associated with each of us until death. Unless preventative measures are taken as a person ages, the amount of available Qi diminishes. This often results in such characteristic features of old age as brittle bones, an increasing rigidity in the skeletal and muscular structures, less than robust health, a diminished sense of well-being, reduced amounts of energy, and ultimately illness.

Each of us, however, is capable of acquiring and nurturing personal Qi. A nonpractitioner is basically restricted as to the amount of available personal Qi. The total amount and quality depends on exactly what was transmitted at birth. We can all supplement personal Qi depending on our individual nature and capacity. Normally we absorb essential elements from food, drink, and from the air we breathe. Combined with the habits of our daily lives, such as exercise, meditation or prayer, and personal habits, this sums up our attempt at preserving health and strength. The Qi Gong practitioner takes the nutritional process one step further by absorbing Universal Qi directly from nature and transmuting it into life-supporting personal Qi.

The practice of Qi Gong reinforces already existing quantities of prenatal Qi and increases our capacity to store and transmit this vital force. This helps ensure robust health in ourselves, and through its transmission, in others we treat. Although we are all born with the Qi Gong ability, special development is not possible overnight. As the Master from Beijing once remarked on this topic, "According to an ancient Chinese proverb, Rome was not built in a day." He continued by noting that with determination each of us is capable of mastering the practice.

QI OF NATURE

According to Chinese tradition, the Qi of Nature created both the 10,000 things and human life. Qi works throughout all of nature to ensure growth and evolution. Without it, life would not exist. In classical Indian philosophy, Qi is referred to as Prana. It is described in Yogi Ramacharaka's book, *The Hindu-Yogi Science of Breath,* as a universal principle, the essence or soul of all force, motion and energy. According to Ramacharaka, although it exists in matter and in air, it is composed of a finer, more vital essence, and permeates virtually everything. Mastering the science of storing away Prana infuses the practitioner with vitality and strength which can be felt by others. The phenomenon of magnetic healing is effected in this way.[2]

Our own discipline, Qi Gong, teaches people to exercise in ways that specifically permit prenatal Qi to develop and strengthen. Over time, practitioners will regain a natural "tightness" about their bodies. This tension promotes better health, allows the development of more sophisticated personal faculties, and ultimately leads to a more complete worldview.

In Traditional Chinese Medicine, it is a well-established principle that the blood in the body follows the Qi. This means that the circulation in the body is dependent upon and reflects the flow of Qi. Regular practice of Qi Gong promotes the flow of Qi, whose presence, in turn, will attract and guide the blood. This relationship strengthens the entire body.

For the most part, the average individual is not fully aware of Qi, either as it appears in the body, or in the natural world around us. Since it is the most fundamental of all elements, it operates at the root of our experience. Qi is the substance that informs all other lesser elements. Since it operates below the threshold of modern consciousness, we are generally unaware of its presence and cannot detect its subtle, though commanding, influences.

Some aboriginal people still seem to have close, direct contact with this force. Recognizing this helps to account for such strange feats among these people as telepathy, shamanic healing, and precognition. With practice, we can all reawaken our ability to recognize and use this force. Since Qi is the primary characteristic of living things, it is our heritage to be familiar with all of its properties. Unfortunately, modern living has blunted our senses to the point where they no longer are capable of identifying Qi. As a result of the predominance of empirical methodology in science, the Western world has not had much room in either its philosophical or psychological theory for such a concept. After all, according to

---

2. Yogi Ramacharaka, *The Hindu-Yogi Science of Breath* (London: L.N. Fowler, Ltd., 1960), pp. 18-22.

the science of the day, the Qi cannot be touched, or seen, or felt, and we have never even been able to measure it with our instruments. With this mass of evidence to the contrary, the argument runs, how could a substance like Qi possibly exist?

Kirlian photography is one instrument which allows us to make these measurements. The technique clearly demonstrates a strange radiation emanating from living tissues, whether they are plant or animal in origin. Interestingly, the ancient texts from India and elsewhere, some written 5,000 years ago or more, clearly describe the same phenomenon, sometimes in vivid detail. It is no accident that these passages use terms such as luminous, glowing, light, or shining to describe the Qi. Far more than any other characteristic, Qi can be identified most readily as a form of light. In fact, it can be conceived of as the embodiment of light.

The Sanskrit word "veda" means wisdom or science. In a general sense, though, it is the term ascribed to the ancient literature of India. Some of these writings predate the Christian era by several millennia. The following dialogue, from *The Upanishads: Breath of the Eternal*, is one of the principal Vedic texts. The passage describes the inner aspects of a practitioner or devotee as seen by the instructor:

> *In due time Satyakama returned home. When he saw Upakosala, he said: "My son, your eyes shine like one who knows Brahman. Who has taught you?*
>
> *"Beings other than men," replied Upakosala.*
>
> *Then said Satyakama: "My son, what you have learned is true. True also is this that I teach you now. Lo, to him who knows it no evil shall cling, even as drops of water cling not to the leaf of the lotus."*
>
> *"He who glows in the depths of your eyes — that is Brahman; that is the Self of yourself. He is the Beautiful One, he is the Luminous One. In all worlds, forever and ever, he shines."*[3]

---

3. Swami Prabhavananda and Frederick Manchester, trans., *The Upanishads: Breath of the Eternal* (New York: Signet, 1975), pp. 67, 68.

Several thousands of years later, sometime in the third century A.D., a similar observation is expressed in *The Bhagavad Gita*, one of the central texts of Hinduism. This passage is interpreted by Yogi Ramacharaka.

> *I see thee with crown of Universal Glory, armed with the Universal weapons of mighty power. And darting from Thee on all sides, I see wondrous beams of effulgent radiance and glorious brilliancy. Difficult it is to see Thee at all, for the light, like unto the rays of a million-million suns, multiplied and magnified a million-million times, dazzleth even the divine eye with which thou has endowed me."[4]*

Until the recent technological breakthrough in Kirlian photography, the privilege of seeing the energy field of the Qi has been reserved only for a special few. After comparing the descriptions in the ancient passages written by one of the ancients with a Kirlian photograph, it is an easy matter to see that the photograph and the text describe similar if not identical phenomena.

Without any formal training, young children have the best sense of Qi and its uses. In these early ages, intellectual training has not yet interfered with or damaged the intuitive faculties. Even in the early stages of our cognitive development, we are still able to recognize this force and actually put it to use. One obvious use is the remarkable ability of children to learn. In hindsight it is difficult to appreciate the volume of information children must learn simply to interact in a successful manner with their world.

Another constructive insight into the nature of Qi is the fact that values and attitudes acquired in youth, when the Qi is strongest, generally remain with us for the duration of our lives. It may be that the Qi actually heightens our emotions or is their source, thereby giving us youthful and powerful associations with events. This would explain the obstinacy with which notions acquired in younger years remain with us, often defying reasoned judgment. It would also explain why it is so difficult for older peo-

---

4. Yogi Ramacharaka, *The Bhagavad Gita* (Chicago: The Yogi Publication Society, 1907), p. 113.

ple to accept new ideas or ways of behavior— simply put, Qi is unavailable in old age.

Rare individuals have one or more special talents which enable them to see or sense the Qi through some unusual faculty. Some of us, for example, can clearly see the Qi appearing in the air as tiny globes or spirals of light. Others feel it in the palms of their hands as it emanates from living tissues such as the petals of flowers or the bark of a tree. As we age, our ability to sense Qi begins to diminish. Regular practice of specific exercises can reawaken our sensitivity to it. This enables us to detect its presence or absence in ourselves or in the environment and to use it for various purposes. Once we develop this skill, we are better able to attract it, to store it, and to process it. Eventually we can also emit it in significant quantities.

THE FUNCTIONS OF QI

Qi pervades all living bodies. It is even present in what we consider inanimate objects, to a greater or lesser extent depending on the qualities of the substance itself. In the human body, it is distributed in individual organs, groups of organs, tissues or other structures. Because of its primacy and the central role it plays in all activities, the brain, for example, requires proportionately greater amounts of Qi than other organs to function efficiently.

Gopi Krishna, in his spellbinding book, *Living with Kundalini*, chronicles the effects of increased quantities of Qi on the brain. Page after page, he takes the reader on a rarely paralleled adventure into the unknown reaches of the human mind. Both the style and content of his book reflect three qualities of the enlightened mind: elegance, simplicity, and clarity in speech. With superb technique, he reveals the dramatic mysteries and workings of Prana or Qi, as it affects both our physiology and our psychology.

There are many different subtypes of Qi, but in our daily practice, we are only concerned with three. The Whei Qi, or Guarding Qi, circulates near the skin, outside the channels. It is primarily a Yang or masculine energy. Whei Qi is produced from the Yang Qi generated in the kidneys. It then moves into the central body area between the navel and the diaphragm. This is known as the Central Heater or Central Burner. There it uses the Qi produced by the spleen and the stomach to support it as it moves into the area above the diaphragm known as the Upper Burner, where it is further developed by the lungs.

Its purpose, as explained in the ancient texts, is described in the following way: Whei Qi is fast moving and slippery. It does not enter the channels, but circulates in the skin and muscles. It is primarily distributed in the chest and belly. Whei Qi functions to keep one warm and to keep the skin flexible and moist. In a general sense, it gives one strength and controls the opening and closing of the acupuncture points.

A contemporary description of Whei Qi says that it nurses the channels, keeps the skin healthy, and opens and closes the pores. It acts as a protective agent against germs and "evil" Qi. It underlies the functioning of the immune system and is strong and slippery in nature. When the Whei Qi is flowing properly, as it tends to do during waking hours, it is difficult to fall ill. When we sleep, however, and the Whei Qi is not circulating as freely, it is easier to succumb to certain diseases.

Yin Qi, or Nutritional Qi, circulates around the internal organs and the channels. This Qi is described as Yin since it resides internally rather than on the surface. Both Whei Qi and Yin Qi are transformed into each other during their circuitous route through the body. Both are created from the food we eat, the liquids we drink, and the air we breathe.

According to the ancients, Yin Qi controls salivation, sweating, digestive juices, and all fluid functions of the body. It travels along the channels in a passive, obedient manner and, in addition to assisting in the process of growth, it nurses the internal organs, and cleans the six Yin channels; three of these channels are associated with the hands and another three with the feet.

Qi of the Internal Organs and Channels consists of five different Qi essences which function to strengthen and preserve the organs and their operations. These types of Qi cannot be emitted, but reside permanently in the organs and channels. Together they maintain homeostasis in the body and give strength to the immune system. Continuing life depends upon these Qi essences.

THE BLOOD AND
ITS RELATIONSHIP TO QI

Chinese medical theory maintains that the blood is created by the functioning of the organs in the Triple Burner, primarily the stomach, liver, and spleen. It is clear that the ancients understood the fundamental importance of blood. An expression from antiquity explains that "once the liver is supplied with blood, then we can see; once the feet are supplied with blood, then we can walk; once the hands are supplied with blood, then we can grasp." After recognizing the essential character of both blood and Qi, and the many parallels between them, it was an easy step for practitioners to conceive of these two substances as existing within a symbiotic relationship.

The truth of this ancient observation can be demonstrated using a simple Chinese technique for strengthening the hands and fingers, thereby improving the blood flow and the circulation. Baoding balls, also known as exercise balls, are two hollow steel balls with small pieces of metal floating about inside. This feature enables the balls to ring with a pleasing sound as they are rolled. In a pair, one ball rings high and the other low. They are made in various sizes to suit different palms, and the precise effect they will have on your hands depends on the type you use.

After sufficient practice, the hands and fingers will gain strength and dexterity. Some Baoding balls are solid and extremely heavy. After several months of using this type, your hands will gain enormous strength. Using the hollow type, the hands and fingers become very nimble. Eventually, the finger tips are permeated with enough Qi to pick up or manipulate the tiniest of objects. Such an exercise is useful for musicians, artists, and others who need to use their hands in precise ways.

The organs, limbs, and brain all require blood to function. Tradition has it that while Qi is the leader and director (Yang) of the blood, the blood is the mother (Yin) of Qi. As a result of this relationship, the two substances are completely interdependent. When the Qi is circulating, then the blood will also be circulating. If the Qi is blocked, then the blood will stop flowing properly and pain or pathological conditions will develop in that location.

An accurate understanding of Qi and its functions requires extensive study of Traditional Chinese Medicine. Those who have some knowledge of the various channels and acupuncture points will use the methods of Qi Gong with the most success. One text, *The Web that has No Weaver*, by Ted J. Kaptchuk, is a thorough and reliable primer in this mysterious discipline. Regardless of how many books are consulted, though, the mysteries of Qi can never be fully understood without actual practice.

THE STUDY OF QI — A FRONTIER SCIENCE

In China, Qi Gong is regarded as a frontier science because its results defy beliefs commonly held in the scientific community. As we become more aware of this natural force, we will be able to use hitherto untapped resources. As in any discipline, dedication to the art will enable us to develop special and often unusual talents. Abilities, such as seeing events and hearing sounds thousands of miles away, using a type of x-ray vision to see inner anatomical structures, exhibitions of exceptional strength, and displays of telekinesis are regarded as commonplace by practioners of the discipline.

At this point in time, these extraordinary body senses and functions are not fully understood, not even by the Qi Gong Masters themselves. Even Western science, highly refined in some ways, does not understand the human body, or the processes involved with life itself, well enough to explain the unusual phenomena associated with Qi Gong. As a result of this inability to deal with the phenomenon using traditional terms, a new word, *bioinformation*, has been coined in China. The term refers to the type of information specifically related to the body and to its inner processes.

Since our prehistoric origins and even early on in the modern age, we have had to rely on special senses and abilities simply to survive. During the shift from hunting and gathering as a way of life, to farming and industrial occupations, we lost touch with the physical world around us. As a result, we no longer had to deal directly with other forms of life. We lived and worked essentially in isolation, interacting only with ourselves and the constructions we built. Our senses of smell and hearing diminished, and our overall sensitivity to the natural world declined.

Our artificial world now extends into both the physical and psychic realms. While this environment shelters us from natural forces, we also have lost the opportunity to bathe in starlight and to breathe deeply in the presence of the full moon. And so, over the last eight thousand years or so, our special senses have deteriorated to the point where they are no longer apparent in the modern person. This does not mean that these features cannot be reawakened, but only that their appearance in the average person is unusual and considered abnormal.

Although these abilities are largely lost, or in a latent state, in our contemporary world, they can be considered as very advanced qualities which have degenerated through lack of use. These senses have been referred to as extrasensory perceptions. Unfortunately, these qualities are often denigrated as the preposterous illusions of madmen or charlatans by those who presume themselves to be knowledgeable in matters of what is and what is not real. This primitive attitude has the ultimate effect of undermining individual experience, and delaying the organization of scientific research into these special categories of human experience.

According to the Qi Gong Masters themselves, there are many special talents. For example, they speak of the five supernatural powers. *Deva Vision* and *Deva Hearing* are the abilities to see and hear events thousands of miles away, or even in other dimensions. *Other's Heart* is the ability to know the innermost thoughts of others. *Tell Life* is the facility to see into past lives. *Travel Beyond* is the skill which enables travel into the astral planes. When all of these abilities are combined in one person, the individual enters into the *League of Beings Above and Beyond Commoners.*

The goal of Shaolin Nei Jin Qi Gong, though, is not necessarily to develop powers such as these, but to develop only those abilities specifically suited for healing. As the Master from Beijing expressed it, "If the ability does not help me with my practice, I am not interested."

While there are other benefits, the central purpose of the exercises described in the subsequent pages is to assist the practitioner in reawakening and strengthening latent abilities common to all human beings for the purpose of healing self and others.

ORIGINS OF QI GONG

Qi Gong, in its original form, may be as much as 4,500 years old. There are many theories as to how it came into the world. It may have originated through experimentation by individuals attempting to heal themselves, their family, or friends, by stimulating various points of the body. It may also have been the work of a single genius who, cloistered somewhere in a monastery, noticed odd relationships between postures and physical well-being. Some also believe the art to have divine origins. Whatever its source, it has been the major preoccupation of innumerable devotees for thousands of years. Entering into this discipline conjoins you to this silent brotherhood.

The art, itself, has historically been passed on through the generations in secret traditions. While there are esoteric reasons for secrecy, there are also very practical ones. Chinese emperors, for example, have had a habit of persecuting monks, particularly Taoists, and have harassed, imprisoned, tortured, and murdered them, and burned their books regularly and with impunity. For the time being, though, it is reasonably safe to practice, and secrecy is not strictly necessary, unless it is to preserve certain practices from public scrutiny.

The central premise of Qi Gong is that the discipline has the capacity to unify (or perhaps reunify) human beings with heaven.

Just as the universe itself is complete, so is human life. We are born into a cycle, often symbolized as a wheel. Our birth is an entry point into the mortal aspects of that cycle. We all move from birth to death through the stages common to human existence. As we mature, we encounter various states of sickness and health on the way.

Traditional Chinese Medicine (TCM) focuses on the treatment of specific ailments. Qi Gong is only one dimension of TCM. Its practice induces harmony between the body and mind, making us more sensitive to physical requirements for a long and healthy life. This quality of knowledge puts the mind and body in the best possible relationship.

Another group of historically significant TCM theorists were the nutritionists, a divergent group of medical practitioners who moved away from the notion of treating specific diseases, preferring instead a holistic view of the patient. Eventually, they focused their attention on the problem of longevity. Both groups, however, attended to the process of living, and were very interested in studying the human body in its daily operations. As a result, nutritionists have always held a close relationship with the discipline of Qi Gong. In their practice, nutritionists consider three elements common to all human beings: Jing or essence, Qi or vital energy, and Shen or spirit.

From the writings generally attributed to Lao Tsu, the Taoist monk and philosopher, presumably a contemporary of K'ung Fu-Tsu, known in the West as Confucius, we can see ample evidence that he was well aware of the inner nature of Qi Gong. In fact, during his life, Qi Gong was refined to a high art. The monk himself recommended cultivating a modest and quiet heart, a relaxed and peaceful body, and a mind without desire. Achieving this, he maintained, only required that we "be natural." What exactly he meant by this has been the subject of much discussion over the centuries. These characteristics are outlined in more detail in his treatise, *The Tao Te Ching*.[5] Following his own advice, something most of us are simply unable to do, he reputedly lived to be 160 years old.

---

5. A modern translation of *The Tao Te Ching* is available by Stephen Mitchell (New York: Harper Perennial, 1991).

K'ung Fu-Tsu had 3,000 students, including 72 Masters of the six arts (ceremonies, music, archery, carriage driving, writing, and mathematics). He said that a statesman or an intellectual should first of all take care of the body, secondly run the country, and only lastly attempt to conquer the world. The implication is that the physical body is the foundation for successful action in the world.

Buddhism was carried into China during the Han Dynasty, about A.D. 2, from its place of origin in India. Chan Buddhism, which means calm or peaceful consideration, has evolved along two philosophical lines: one of sitting and one of realizing or prolonged, intensive practice. Both forms cultivate a spiritual dimension, and both can lead to psycho-physiological changes in the body. This connection to spirit is one reason Qi Gong is often associated with Buddhism. For some practitioners, Buddhism offers an intellectual and spiritual foundation for the practice of Qi Gong.

Just as Qi Gong has benefited from its association with Buddhism over the centuries, so other disciplines, such as calligraphy, the martial arts, and acupuncture have profited from their association with Qi Gong. In fact, this has so often been the case that Qi Gong is frequently thought of as a means to improve another practice, rather than as a distinct practice complete with its own goals.

Our form of this art, Shaolin Nei Jin Qi Gong, was originally a secret tradition passed on by a wandering Indian monk, Da Mo, later called Bodhidharma. Born in A.D. 440, in Kanchi, the capital of the southern Indian Kingdom of Pallava, he is now venerated as the one who brought these meditation techniques to China. Bodhidharma is also considered to be the founder of Chan Buddhism, known also by its Japanese equivalent of Zen.

Late in the fifth century, he traveled to China from India. During this period of Chinese history, two rival empires existed, the Northern Wei and the Liu Sung Dynasties. After meeting with Emperor Wu of the Liang Dynasty (successor to the Liu Sung Dynasty) who did not understand his teachings, he left the region for the North. Eventually, he moved into the Shaolin temple on the sacred mountain, Mount Sung. Ironically, this temple was built by the Emperor Hsiao-wen for another Indian meditation Master whose name has since been forgotten.

Many legends persist about Da Mo, one being that he lived 150 years. Other stories find him performing the Horse Stance while facing a wall of a cave for nine years. He also taught early forms of martial arts and preached Chan Buddhist doctrine. Some of his works still survive. In his book, *The Zen Teachings of Bodhidharma,* Red Pine translates four of these: *Outline of Practice, The Blood Stream Sermon, The Wake Up Sermon,* and *The Breakthrough Sermon.*

Since the temple at that time was not large, he practiced in a nearby cave, as did his successors. This allowed for a great deal of secrecy, and because the temple rules were very strict, the various Qi Gong techniques and specific information were never passed on to outsiders, but only to selected monks. Until recently, in fact, very few people in China, itself, knew anything about Shaolin Nei Jin Qi Gong.

MODERN HISTORY

Shaolin Nei Jin Qi Gong is known as a soft or healing form. Since its methods rely on intensive physical practice, it is also a realizing form. This Gong is also referred to as the One-Finger Gong. Its odd nickname is derived from the technique of emitting Qi from the fingertips. Typically, this serves the purpose of treating the physical ailments of others.

The practice has been called the One-Finger Chan, as well. This form became famous as a result of the exploits of a Chinese monk, Hai Den, still alive in 1988. He was able to rest the entire weight of his body on one finger. As an octogenarian, the monk is reputed to have traveled to the United States to demonstrate this remarkable ability.

The specific techniques discussed later in the text are derived directly from the teachings of Que Ahshui, a monk who was born in 1926 near Shanghai. His family was poor, and when he entered a Shaolin temple, hard-practice Qi Gong was the main discipline.

He was assigned the menial tasks of sweeping the floor, topping off the oil lamps, dusting the statues, carrying water, and the like. For a Buddhist, this type of assignment is not considered unfortunate. The monk believes that hard labor in this life, without complaint or regret, will bring an easier life in the next incarnation.

The monk Dush Umbio undertook to instruct Que Ahshui and taught him both the realizing form of Shaolin Nei Jin Qi Gong and the martial arts. Subsequently, he worked as a sweeper in Shanghai. For many years, he remained virtually unknown for his exceptional abilities. When he miraculously cured someone with a serious medical condition, the government requested that he write a book on the topic. Unfortunately, during the cultural revolution, he was imprisoned and, as a result of the hardships he endured, he died an early death in 1978. The person he healed, however, became Que Ahshui's successor and as of 1987 was still alive.

FOUR UNIQUE FEATURES OF SHAOLIN NEI JIN QI GONG

1. Infinite Energy

In China there are more than 3,000 styles of Qi Gong. Among these, there are many prescriptions as to how best to develop the Qi. The techniques include methods for concentrating on certain parts of the body or energy centers. Principal of these centers is the Shimen, also known as the Tantien point. The Shimen is a point well-known in the martial arts. Found approximately one-and-a-half inches below the navel, and an equal distance inward, it is regarded as the epicenter of the body. In other practices, meditations are typically used, together with postures, to concentrate the Qi in this region.

Exotic Qi Gong techniques which rely on the Shimen point are used for innumerable purposes. Some methods relax body and mind, seek to improve circulation, or increase the quality and quantity of available Qi. Still others have their focus on moving the

Qi more efficiently through the body, or enable its transmission to others.

With our form, however, we disregard all prescriptions using the Shimen point (with the exception of the Awakening the Heavenly Eye: Form 2 Meditation). It is neither necessary for us to become meditation Masters, nor to use exotic breathing techniques. It is only important to relax and to maintain correct posture when doing the exercises. Talking to others, listening to the radio, or even watching television when practicing is perfectly acceptable, and even encouraged. While it is a difficult concept for many people to accept, concentration or meditation is not necessary. The body has a wisdom of its own and does not always require the conscious intervention of the mind for direction. The Qi develops on its own accord as a result of the postures we assume. In fact, concentration can actually diminish the results of practice.

There is another reason we avoid meditation during these exercises. The Master from Beijing stated on more than one occasion that "entering the silence" (meditating while practicing) has been known to produce dangerous energy imbalances. This unbalanced state, he continued, can only be rectified, if at all, by an experienced Master. So, when practicing, keep your eyes open, and your mind relaxed and preoccupied.

Shaolin Nei Jin Qi Gong will enable us to treat patients all day long without tiring. The reason for this exceptional level of strength is that our training is specifically designed to enable us to collect, transform, and emit universal energy. With proficiency, you will be able to absorb and emit simultaneously. Other forms do not empower the practitioner to this level. One reason for this is that other forms depend on Qi that has been previously stored in the body. Overexertion in these other forms is common, and can deplete your vital energy or lead to serious bodily damage.

2. The Buddhist Light

The practical purposes of Shaolin Nei Jin Qi Gong are to treat patients and to heal self. Healing requires an ability to collect and transform universal energy and then to apply it. Time and again, when speaking of Christ and his miraculous ability to heal, the biblical Gospels refer to this or some similar power. Since there are numerous accounts of Christ leaving populated places for the wilderness, there is little doubt that after using his power, Christ did feel some need to recuperate and replenish his energies. The obvious place for him to do this was in solitude. As well as feeling the need to commune with the divine, he also had to restore his reserves of Qi.

Qi Gong is an art devoted to restoring this divine energy. Throughout the body, there are special places where Universal Qi can most easily enter and leave the body. These places are termed "Qi gates." In time, perhaps with the help of a Master, practitioners will open their Qi gates. In the hand alone, there are more than 20 such gates. Using these gates, large quantities of energy can be collected for processing and storage by the body and later emitted as healing rays. Many people, even without special training, can readily feel these rays as a tingling sensation in the palm or wrist. Practice will heighten this sensation until the presence of Qi is unmistakable.

Internal Qi, or Qi stored in the body, is also called Real Qi. When it is emitted, it is referred to as External Qi. After some practice, it is possible to collect energy and emit it simultaneously. During the first three months of practice, students should limit the duration and frequency of treatments to one patient a day for 15 or 20 minutes. This will prevent excessive demands on the body.

After many years of practice, the entire body will be filled with light and will be surrounded by an aura which is referred to as the Buddhist Light. There is an interesting reference in one of the Gospels which refers to this light. Christ says, "If thine eye be single, thy whole body will be filled with light."

The reference here is to the Heavenly Eye, commonly known as the Third Eye. According to esoteric literature, this eye will only awaken at a certain level of spiritual purity and awareness. Is Christ referring in the passage to the advanced spiritual insights generated by an awakened consciousness and represented by the Heavenly Eye? Qi Gong practitioners understand this message as

an indirect reference which pertains to the opening of certain channels in the body. This, in turn, permits the Qi to circulate into hitherto inaccessible regions of the brain. This circulation is responsible
for the light, or halo, often reported surrounding saints and holy
people. As the Heavenly Eye awakens, it induces further biochem-
ical reactions in the body which result in a strengthened aura. This
is very often visible to people with heightened senses. Artists, for
example, often depict saints with such a halo. This is not an imag-
ined attribute but one that is very real.

In the intermediate series of Shaolin Qi Gong exercises,
known as the Arhat or Luo Han, there is an exercise designed
specifically to develop this inner light. It is appropriately named
The Buddhist Light. This light acts as a protective force and guards
against illness. When your body emits the light on a regular basis,
perhaps after two or three years of consistent practice, the frequency and duration of treatments can be as long as necessary.

3. Bending-Finger Method

The Bending-Finger Method is the central technique in this style of
Qi Gong. It is unique to Shaolin Nei Jin Qi Gong, and it is the key
to successful practice. As a result of an unusually high density of
nerves and acupuncture points, the fingertips naturally have a
great deal of Qi which flows along six channels, three on the Yin
(palm) side and three on the Yang (top) side. Perfectly round,
palm-sized balls called Baoding balls are often used to exercise the
palm and fingertips. Another finger exercise was offered by the
Master from Shanghai. When shown the Baoding balls, he looked
scornfully at them, made two fists, and flicked his fingers forceful-
ly a dozen times, indicating his preferred way of moving Qi
through fingers.

The fingertips are connected with internal organs which we
exercise during the bending-finger movements. When we bend the
fingers, we are soothing and curing the associated internal organs.
The thumb, for example, is associated through a channel with the
lungs. If some problem with a lung develops, the thumb is bent in

a special manner, a certain number of times, for a set duration, and in a certain sequence. Depending on the nature of the illness, the thumb is sometimes bent in association with other fingers. In this way the practitioner promotes the flow of health-giving Qi to the lungs.

4. State of Mind

There are many techniques which allow the practice of Qi Gong in different circumstances. We can be standing, sitting, lying down, or walking when we practice. Age or sex makes no difference, although it is unusual to find children practicing seriously. What is important is our state of mind. When we are still and calm, we are nourishing our Qi. When we move, we are using our Qi. When practicing, remember that the mind can be still when the body moves. This gives rise to a paradox: there can be stillness in movement and movement in stillness.

CHAPTER 2

The Discipline

As discussed earlier, above all the practitioner should cultivate a lifestyle conducive to success. The single most influential quality in this lifestyle is regularity in daily affairs. Aristotle (384-322 B.C.) succinctly articulated this predicament in his Theory of the Golden Mean. Moderation in all things, he maintained, was the key to all good things.

Whatever else you decide to do, you will have to find specific times during the day when you can practice without interruption. By doing this, you will save yourself much grief, and you will soon master the basic techniques. Remember that the effects of Qi Gong are cumulative and that steady practice every day is infinitely superior to long, arduous practice occasionally.

There are a number of habits which detract from a flourishing practice. These are listed below in no particular order:

- Eating or drinking too much or too little;
- Sleeping or working too much;
- Irregular hours of rising and sleeping;
- Being excited and loud in one's daily dealings;
- Excessive emotional absorption in personal relationships;
- Regular consumption of spicy, rich foods;
- Working throughout the night;
- Excesses in general, including sexual practice.

It is important not to practice on either an empty or a full stomach. Doing so is harmful, and the exercise itself will be of little benefit. Wait at least an hour after eating a full meal. Qi Gong practice requires a great deal of oxygenated blood which might not be as available if your stomach is full. Too much food in the stomach creates a pressure on the lungs, which in turn inhibits inhalation and exhalation.

Practicing with too little food in the stomach creates a condition in which the body becomes increasingly cold. There is nothing for the body to draw on to replace the vital energy which leaves the hands during practice. This can damage the stomach. Before morning practice, a cup of tea or a glass of milk and some fruit or hot cereal will relieve the hunger.

If you have an ulcer, it is particularly important that you eat something before practice. Also, the food should be warm, not cold, and eaten without a great deal of spice. Excessive amounts of spice or cold food will weaken the body.[1]

It is essential during practice to be very relaxed. This cannot be emphasized strongly enough. Wearing loose fitting clothes, clearing out the bowels beforehand, choosing a scenic view, and ensuring fresh air circulation will do much to promote relaxation and contribute to a healthy state of mind and body.

Beautiful scenery, such as a flowing river or a spot high in the mountains, will allow the creation of Noble or Imperishable Qi. Noble Qi can be described as the difference between the feelings generated in a slum and those in a high alpine meadow.

Never practice in wet, damp, windy, or cold places. Winds from the east and west are not always harmful but those from the north or south can be dangerous. Do not practice near bodies of water if there are strong winds. If you practice indoors, avoid drafts.

Students in good health should practice for one hour a day. This time should be specific, and preferably split evenly between

1. When the Master from Beijing first arrived in North America, he noticed that large amounts of cold Qi had accumulated in the stomach regions of most people he treated. He later realized that the phenomenon was due to the Western habit of placing almost all food in the refrigerator.

morning and evening. The length of practice can be decreased if you suffer from some ailment. If you are physically weak or at a disadvantage, it is better to increase the frequency of practice to four times a day at 15 minutes each, rather than to maintain a one hour practice period.

If you suffer from insomnia, do all your practice in the morning. If you are frequently tired or in a bad mood, if you have mental difficulties, or are excessively emotional, it may not be advisable to practice this form of Qi Gong. You may practice, however, if your condition is stable or if you are under medication.

Women should practice less frequently during menstruation, or, if there are difficulties, stop altogether. If there is no discomfort, there is no reason to stop. Practicing during the first three months of pregnancy is fine, but subsequent practice is inadvisable. Standing in the Horse Stance can be dangerous during pregnancy.

For best results, do not let anyone stand behind you. It is irritating and upsetting to have activities conducted behind one's back. In China and elsewhere there are unscrupulous Masters who are able to steal personal Qi. This repugnant practice is generally performed from behind. The Master from Beijing added that in North America, as of 1987, he had not seen anyone capable of such an act.

For those who practice professionally, it is also better to face directly north or south during practice, and to use light cotton socks or soft leather-soled shoes, such as moccasins. Also, remove rings or other jewelry beforehand, as such items can impede the flow of Qi.

Warm Up Exercises

Warm up exercises are practiced before the four general sets. By performing them, you will improve the flow of the Qi in the body and prepare it for the forthcoming exercises. There are four warm ups, named Grinding the Beans, Making Straw Rope, The Shoulder Pole, and Circle the Shoulder.

Before beginning your practice, here are a few reminders. Remember not to practice in windy or damp places. During Qi Gong exercise, the Qi gates in the body open and Qi is freely exchanged with the surrounding environment. According to ancient tradition, the wind and damp air are notorious for attacking the body, and are especially dangerous at this time.

It is preferable to stand in the light of the stars, moon, or sun. The Qi emitted by these heavenly bodies is beneficial, and during practice we have an opportunity to absorb it. On the other hand, if the sun is too strong, do not face directly into it. The level of energy in the sunlight at these times can be dangerous and can actually "scorch" the interior routes used by the Qi. Since your eyes absorb a great deal of Qi, by facing away from the sun, you can still gain the benefits of Qi from the sun without danger. Finally, remember that it is inadvisable to let people stand directly behind you when you practice this or any similar discipline.

WARM UP NO. I: GRINDING THE BEANS

From a relaxed and comfortable standing posture, take one step forward with the right foot and bend slightly at the right knee. Turn the left foot so that it angles outward at 45 degrees. The right heel should be in line with the left heel. This is called the Arrow Stance.

Place your left hand on the spleen area just over the hip and lean forward. Stretch out your right arm. With the right palm facing the floor, your arm should begin to make a circular motion away from the body so that it describes a full circle. Make 20 circles. Now reverse the direction for another 20 circles so that the hand is moving toward the body.

Do the same thing with the left foot outstretched using your left arm to make the circles. Place your right hand over the liver area. Imagine you are expelling unhealthy Qi from your body when your arms are moving outward. When your arms are moving toward you, imagine absorbing healthy, Universal Qi. Push this healthy Qi into your body with your hand (without actually touching your chest) as it passes by. You should be making these circles with moderate speed and vigor.

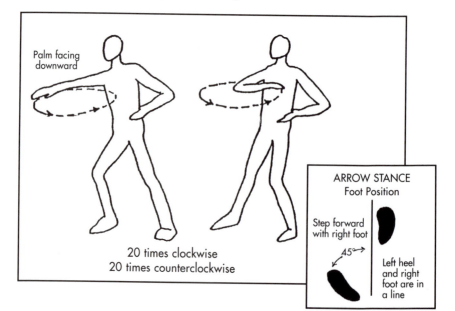

Palm facing downward

20 times clockwise
20 times counterclockwise

ARROW STANCE
Foot Position

Step forward with right foot

45°

Left heel and right foot are in a line

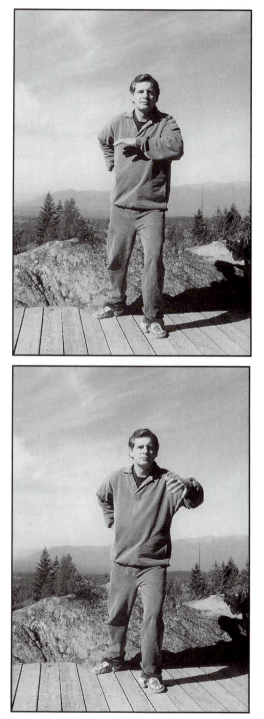

Opening position.

Absorbing healthy
Universal Qi.

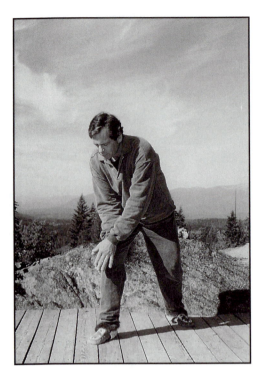

Opening position.

WARM UP NO. 2: MAKING STRAW ROPE

From a standing position, assume the Arrow Stance, right leg forward. Place the back of your right hand, with the palm face up, over your right kneecap. The back of your hand should be touching the knee. This hand remains fixed for the duration of the exercise. It keeps your body in place and ensures that it does not move too far backward. If the hand on the knee moves, the benefits of Making Straw Rope will be lost.

Place your left hand over the right palm so that the fingers line up. Move your left hand up along the inside of your right arm, breathing in as you do so. When your hand reaches your shoulder, trace an arc, lightly touching your chest, directly across the top of your body, past your throat, and down the other side.

Pause when you reach your hip. Now breathe out making a hissing sound and return the left palm to its place over the right palm, which is still in position over the knee. The hissing sound is said to increase the amount of Qi you are emitting. It is used in a number of Qi Gong exercises. As you do this set of movements, you will have to straighten your right leg as your left hand moves up your right arm. As this happens, your left leg, behind you, will naturally bend. Moving forward again, your legs will take their original positions. This results in a forward and backward motion. Repeat this 10 times on each side of your body.

Be certain that the palm of the moving hand lightly touches your body as it traces its arc. In this way, it massages the organs. As you will discover later, a Qi Gong massage is unlike almost any other form of massage, in that it relies entirely on the emission of Qi to effect results. Many other forms depend largely on physical

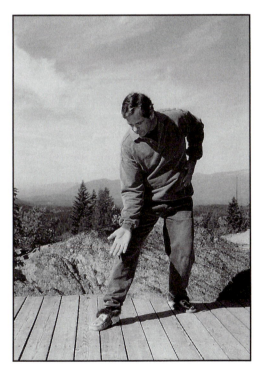

Returning position.

pressure or friction for their results. A Qi Gong massage, on the other hand, is an extremely gentle massage. Since Qi radiates from the palms at the discretion of the practitioner, there is no need to actually massage your client in the traditional sense of the term. The goal of a Qi Gong massage is to push the Qi deep into the body tissues.

In the following exercises, you will occasionally be asked to point your fingers or palms at specific targets on your body. Since Qi radiates from the fingers, you will be replenishing the Qi in specific organs. Certain clothing materials aid in this process while others hinder it. One of the best materials for a patient to wear, or to practice in, is silk. Cotton is another good material. Bare skin, on the other hand, does not conduct Qi very well.

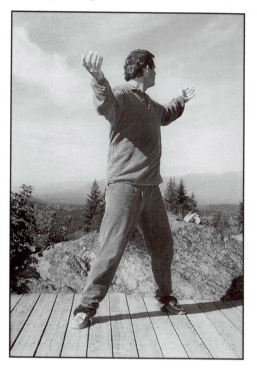

Opening position; looking at
the reference point.

WARM UP NO. 3: SHOULDER POLE

Every so often, looking out from my 11th-floor window, I would see an unusual figure far below running through the university grounds. Resting on his shoulders was a long pole. Two buckets dangled from the ends of the pole. What they contained I never did find out, but that was the first time I saw a shoulder pole in action.

From a standing position, assume the Arrow Stance, left foot forward. Now take a half step back with your right foot. Extend your right arm directly out in front of the body and your left arm behind. Your arms should be slightly bent, not quite as straight as a shoulder pole, and they should remain at shoulder level. Both palms should face to the sky and your knees should be slightly bent as well.

Now turn your head so that you can see behind your body. (Your head can only turn in one direction from this position.)

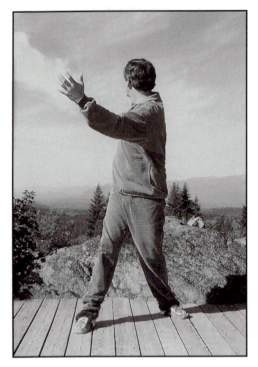

The position nearly reversed.

Choose a spot in the background, one that is directly in line with your left hand. Use this as a reference point. Inhale deeply and swing your arms around from back to front bending several inches at the knees as you do. Make a scooping motion so that the directions of the arms are reversed. Exhale as you move. Straighten the legs as your arms reach their destination.

Your head should follow your arm so that you are now facing the rear wall, looking in a line of sight along your right arm directly at your reference point. After a relaxed count of three, swing your arms back to their original position, making the same scooping motion, inhaling as you move.

This completes one set. Do 10 sets and then reverse your position so that your left foot is forward and out to the side of your body. This time, your left arm should be extended in front and the right behind. Do 10 more sets.

WARM UP NO. 4: CIRCLE THE SHOULDER

This exercise offers a wonderful opportunity to sense the flow of Qi. Close your eyes. Inhale deeply several times and relax completely. From the Natural Stance, move your right arm, palm up, in an arc along the side of your body until it is parallel with your head. Your palm now faces behind you. Turn it around and lower your arm. When you raise your arm, imagine that you are stretching the Qi. When you lower it, imagine that you are compressing it. Many people feel the Qi as a wind or tingling sensation on the palms, and once they become sensitized to it, they actually notice a pressure when they work with it in this way.

The actual exercise is performed as follows. From a standing position, assume the Arrow Stance. Place the palm of your left hand on the spleen area with your thumb on the backside of your

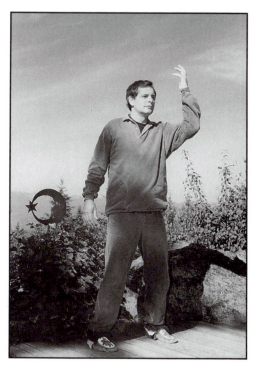

Sensing the Qi: raising the Qi, palm skyward.

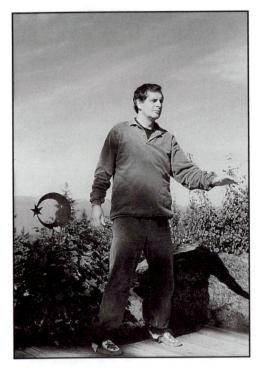

Sensing the Qi: lowering the
Qi, palm earthward.

body. The spleen is located on the left side of the body just below
the diaphragm. Your right arm hangs down by your right side and
the palm of this hand faces to the front of your body. Do this 10
times. Repeat the exercise on the other side of the body.

Be certain that your legs are still, and that your breathing is
natural, during this exercise. The thumb of the moving hand
should be held outstretched. This will open a number of points on
the lung and pericardium channels, activating them in the process.
As a result, your lungs, in particular, will gain strength. This exercise will not work properly if the channel to the lungs is not open.

The First Series

Shaolin Nei Jin Qi Gong has four basic sets. Each set has a number of exercises. In the first set there are four: the Horse Stance, Bending-Fingers, Embracing the Moon with Both Hands, and Holding the Ball with Two Hands. Practitioners generally do all four warm ups, stand for five minutes in the Horse Stance, select one of the two Bending-Finger Methods (two are presented), Embrace the Moon with Both Hands, Hold the Ball with Two Hands, and close the first set with another five minute Horse Stance.

THE HORSE STANCE

There are a number of variations of this common stance, but all have a common purpose: it is used to collect universal energy. Usually it is performed before other exercises are attempted so that the Qi will have already started to move in the channels. This is also true for many of the advanced postures not presented in this text. The Horse Stance is also used as a warm-up exercise. Although it looks simple, it is quite complicated to master. Since it is the cornerstone of all subsequent exercises, perseverance will only benefit your practice.

In the Shaolin Nei Jin version of this stance, stand with both feet together. Now move the left foot one step apart, so that your feet are approximately shoulder-width distance. Initially your arms should be resting at the sides of your body. Raise your arms, palms facing, until they reach waist level. When the palms face each other, they are referred to as "communicating with each other" or "exchanging Qi." After the palms have communicated for a few moments, turn them face down, parallel to the floor, and move your arms in a sweeping arc in front of you, breathing in as you do. Extend your arms to their full length out to the sides of your body.

Now, bend your fingers under your wrists so that they are pointing at your kidneys. Remember that your fingers are capable of emitting Qi. Bring your hands, fingers still directed to the sides, in toward the body at kidney level. As you do this, slowly exhale. Exhaling at this point helps you to emit Qi. A slow, controlled hissing sound is superior to simply letting your breath out with a sigh or a wheeze.

Just before your fingers touch the sides of the body, turn them out to the front, palms still up. When your arms are outstretched to just over half of their full extent, turn the palms down. At the same time, bend slightly at the knees to a point flush with, but not past, your toes. Now move your heels out so that your toes point slightly inward. This movement opens the Changqiang acupuncture point No. 1 on the Du Channel (chapter 5: page 160) , enabling you to accumulate Universal Qi and move it through your body.

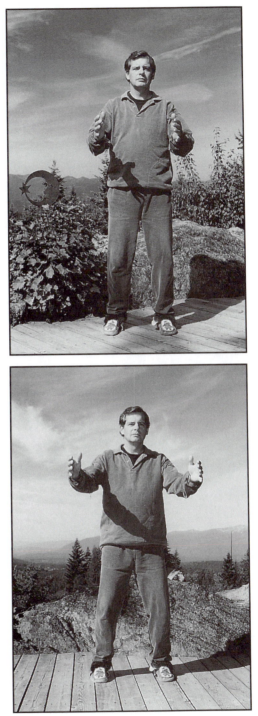

Raising the hands: two
palms communicating.

Hands begin to move apart.

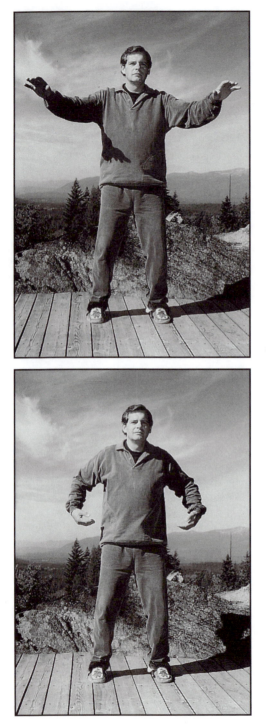

Arms nearly outstretched.

Fingers after emitting Qi to the kidney region.

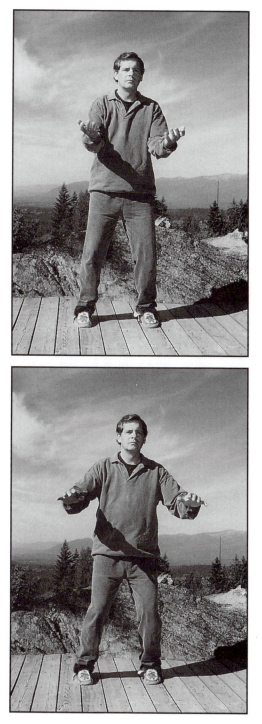

Bring hands to the front, palms skyward.

Hands to the front, knees bending.

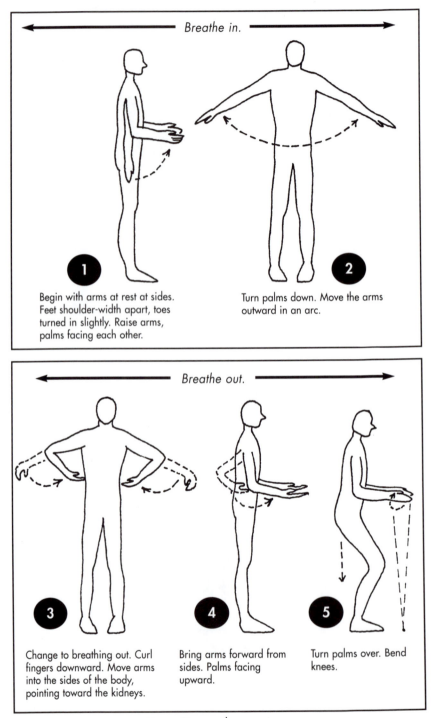

Breathe in.

1 Begin with arms at rest at sides. Feet shoulder-width apart, toes turned in slightly. Raise arms, palms facing each other.

2 Turn palms down. Move the arms outward in an arc.

Breathe out.

3 Change to breathing out. Curl fingers downward. Move arms into the sides of the body, pointing toward the kidneys.

4 Bring arms forward from sides. Palms facing upward.

5 Turn palms over. Bend knees.

Horse Stance: the opening.

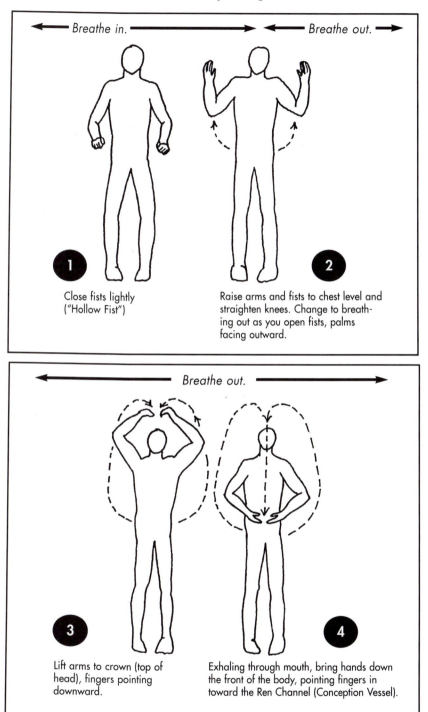

Breathe in. ⟶ ⟵ Breathe out. ⟶

1 Close fists lightly ("Hollow Fist")

2 Raise arms and fists to chest level and straighten knees. Change to breathing out as you open fists, palms facing outward.

⟵ Breathe out. ⟶

3 Lift arms to crown (top of head), fingers pointing downward.

4 Exhaling through mouth, bring hands down the front of the body, pointing fingers in toward the Ren Channel (Conception Vessel).

Horse Stance: the closing.

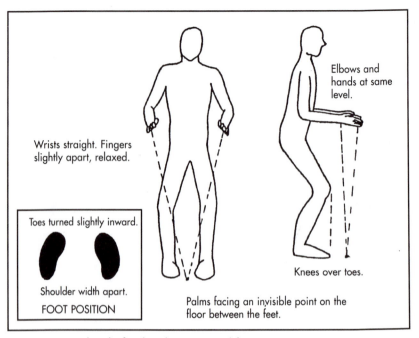

Horse Stance: detail of palm alignment and foot position.

Hold your palms at a slightly inward angle. Imagine two lines drawn from the Laogong point near the center of the palm (chapter 5: page 148) meeting at ground level. If you like, visualize both palms emitting a beam of light which intersects at this spot.

As in all subsequent exercises, it is especially important that your shoulders, neck, and thigh muscles remain relaxed while performing the Horse Stance. Your fingers, wrists, arms, and legs should also be relaxed. Your eyes should be looking straight ahead. Breathe naturally and do not meditate, concentrate, or combine other Qi Gong exercises with the Horse Stance. As soon as the muscles begin to constrict, the pathways used by the Qi will be blocked and the Qi will stop flowing. If this happens, all subsequent exercise is useless. At this point, it may be advantageous to step out of position momentarily to relax and prevent further constriction of your muscles.

Generally, the stance should be held for at least five minutes. After some practice, you can hold it for 30 minutes or more. Later on, experiment with this stance by moving the arms to greater or

lesser distances from the sides of the body. In these different positions, notice the different "frequencies" of Qi as it moves around
and through the arms.

When ending this stance, close the fingers without excessive
pressure to make "Hollow Fists" and, breathing in, bend the forearms so that your fists are lifted to chest level. Straighten the knees
simultaneously. Open the palms and lift the arms to a level with
the head. Exhale through your mouth in the same controlled manner as before, making the usual hissing sound. As you do, bring
your hands down over the back of your head, along the front of
your body with the palms facing your chest. Your fingertips should
be pointing directly at the Ren Channel (which follows the center-
line of the front part of the body) as your hands move down from
your head. When your hands reach their lowest level, relax them
and let them fall to the sides. This is the basic exercise.

Understanding some of the principles involved will impart a
better sense of how this exercise is to be performed. Bending at the
knees, having the palms communicate, and raising the forearms
promotes the circulation of Qi in the three Yin channels of the
hands. Partway through this opening to the Horse Stance, at the
point when your fingers point inward to the Dai (or Belt) Channel
at the level of the kidneys, the Qi emitted from the fingers activates
the Qi in the Dai Channel as well as in the Ren and Du Channel
(which follows the center-line of the back.)

All three channels are activated in this way. Since these channels are connected to each other, the flow of Qi throughout the
entire body is encouraged. Pointing the toes inward causes the Qi
to rush up the spinal column through the Du Channel, passing
through the head to the Ren Channel. Then the Qi moves down
into the three Yin and three Yang foot channels.

Since your arms are not completely outstretched but held
partly back, Qi is stored in the shoulders. As you relax your shoulders, the Qi rushes into the fingertips. You may be able to notice
this yourself in the form of numbness, tingling, or other sensations
in your hands.

BENDING-FINGER METHODS FOR LONGEVITY: METHOD NO. 1

Two methods of the Bending-Finger technique for prolonging life, a method completely unique to Shaolin Nei Jin Qi Gong, are presented here. Because there are more than 20 Qi gates on the hand alone, we exercise it using these techniques, so that we can better absorb and transmit Qi. Since this exercise is beneficial for all internal organs, its consistent practice has acquired the reputation for being able to prolong life. If you are only going to practice one exercise, it should be this one.

After performing the Horse Stance for 5 minutes, remain in the stance and bend the fingers of both hands simultaneously in the following sequence. Table 2 indicates the duration of each bend, the number of times you should bend each finger, and the associated channel of each particular finger.

It should take between 7 and 10 seconds to lower a finger and raise the next. One set should take about five minutes. Do five sets and close with a five-minute Horse Stance. As with all finger bend-

Table 2: Finger-Bending Method No. 1.

FINGER	DURATION	FREQUENCY	POLARITY	CHANNEL
First	50 seconds	1	Yang	Large Intestine
Ring	50 seconds	1	Yang	Triple Burner
Thumb	50 seconds	1	Yin	Lungs
Little (top) (underside)	50 seconds	1	Yang Yin	Small Intestine Heart
Middle	50 seconds	1	Yin	Pericardium

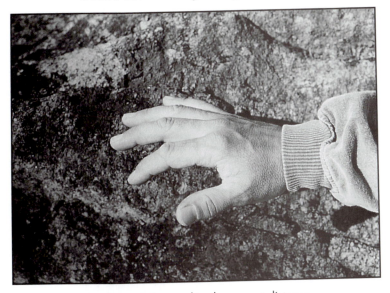

Index finger is lowered to the correct distance.

ing exercises, bend each finger only several centimeters, or about one inch, so that it is not overextended. If you bend your finger too much, the flow of Qi will be blocked. Another point to remember is that when bending the thumb, stretch it outward rather than bending it down. This outward movement has the same effect as bending does on the other fingers.

BENDING-FINGER METHODS FOR LONGEVITY: METHOD NO. 2

After five minutes of the Horse Stance, remain in the stance and bend the fingers in the sequence shown in Table 3 (page 54). For this exercise, the duration includes the time it takes to raise and lower the fingers. This means that the fingers will remain in position between 5 and 7 seconds. Compare the effects of each method. They are very different to perform yet the cumulative effects are similar.

Table 3: Finger-Bending Method No. 2.

FINGER	DURATION	FREQUENCY	POLARITY	CHANNEL
Thumb	8-10 sec	3	Yin	Lungs
Middle	8-10 sec	5	Yin	Pericardium
Small (top)	8-10 sec	3	Yang	Small Intestines
(underside)			Yin	Heart
Index	8-10 sec	7	Yang	Large Intestine
Ring	8-10 sec	9	Yang	Triple Burner
Middle	8-10 sec	1	Yin	Pericardium

After the last finger bend, in this case the middle finger, you have completed one set. Rest for five seconds, still remaining in the Horse Stance and then start again. Do five sets altogether and close with a five-minute Horse Stance. If you feel dizzy during the finger bending or any other of the exercises, sit down and have something to drink before beginning again.

According to Traditional Chinese Medical theory, both your hands and feet are connected to channels. Three of these on each of your hands and feet are Yin and three are Yang in character. Bending a finger causes the Qi to move in a particular channel. This, in turn, sends a signal to the corresponding organ. There are three main benefits from the Bending-Finger exercise: the internal Qi is replenished, the functions of the organs are adjusted, and the circulation of the blood and the Qi is regulated in the entire body. A healthy body and a generous flow of Qi permits external Qi to be emitted in greater amounts and with greater ease.

In chapter 3, we will discuss the various sequences of finger bending which are used in the treatment of specific illnesses.

EMBRACING THE MOON WITH BOTH HANDS

After holding the Horse Stance for five minutes, move your forearms in front of your chest so that both palms face down, and the right palm is above the left elbow. The palm of your right hand is searching for a Qi gate in the elbow. With practice, you will be able to identify this point by feeling a breeze, or soft wind, when your palm passes over it. The sensation is the Qi.

Bend all fingers, including the thumb, on both hands three times, leaving a 1-second gap between bends. (Remember to stretch the thumb outward, rather than down.) Make sure the fingers touch together lightly, making a pear shape. Now inhale and slowly and evenly pull your arms apart, so that the fingers face each other at a distance of two or three inches. There is no need to stretch to your maximum extent, but make sure there is some ten-

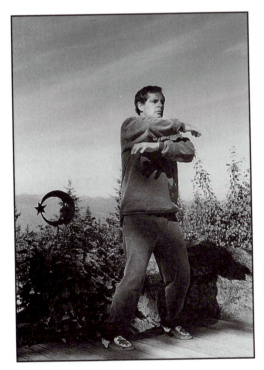

Opening position: palms over elbows before bending fingers.

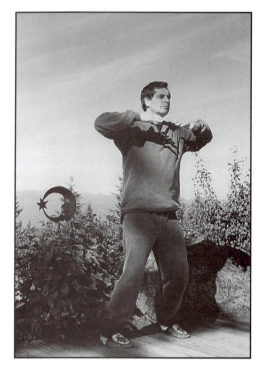

Hands pulling apart: held
for the count of three after
finger-bending.

sion in your shoulders. The degree of tension will differ with the individual.

Hold this position for 3 seconds and then exhale, releasing tension. Push the forearms back to their position, this time with the left palm above the right elbow. Repeat the finger-bending procedures and you will have Embraced the Moon once. Embrace it 10 times altogether. Remember to keep the body relaxed, particularly noting the shoulders, neck, and back muscles.

This exercise is designed to improve the circulation of the Qi in the six channels (three Yin and three Yang) related to the hand. It also adjusts the amount of Qi in both the left and right sides of the body as well as the general balance between the Yin and the Yang Qi throughout the body. Balancing the Qi in this way helps overcome illnesses, particularly respiratory diseases.

HOLDING THE BALL WITH TWO HANDS

From the Horse Stance, cross your forearms, approximately two inches above the wrist crease, with the right on top. Again, as in Embracing the Moon, you are searching for the soft breeze which indicates the flow of Qi. When you feel this breeze, you will have found the correct point for aligning your forearms.

When you find it, pull your arms back so that your right palm is centered over the back of your left hand. The center of your two hands should be aligned. Your hands should be on a level between the solar plexus and the navel, with your thumbs about two or three inches from your body.

With a circling movement, turn your left palm (the bottom hand) over so that it faces and is communicating with your right palm. Inhaling through the nose, draw your hands apart in a vertical motion. This movement stretches or pulls the Qi apart. It is

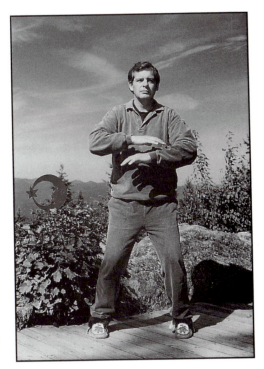

Opening position: palm
aligned over palm.

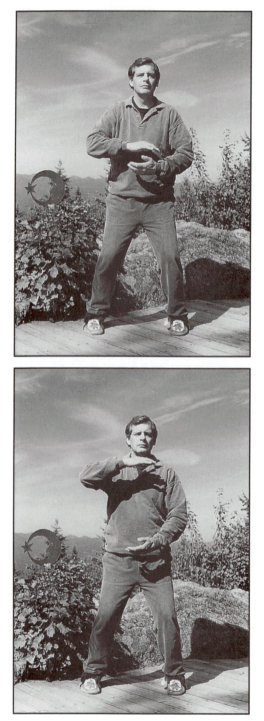

Palms now facing: ready to begin stretching the Qi.

Palms nearly at maximum distance: ready to begin compression of Qi.

important to keep your palms aligned during this motion. Your upper (right) hand should not be raised higher than your forehead while your lower (left) hand should not extend below the groin. At this point, it is time for your hands to begin their return. You do not need to pause here. Exhaling through your mouth, bring your palms back so that they are almost touching. This movement compresses the Qi.

You have now held the ball once. Do 10, and then return to the Horse Stance for one minute. Do 10 more sets with the left palm above, making 20 in all. Since this is the last exercise in this series, close with a five-minute Horse Stance.

When you hold the ball, your palms should look as if they are, in fact, holding a ball. Serious practitioners make a science out of this exercise. For some, the "ball" becomes an indispensable tool. When practicing, you should be able to feel the tension caused by the resistance of the Qi as your hands are moved together and apart.

The mechanical actions of the hands causes the expansion and contraction of the Qi. By pulling the hands apart along the Ren Channel, many acupuncture points are stimulated. This, in turn, stimulates the circulation of Qi in the Ren Channel and as a consequence, the functions of many organs will be adjusted. Diseases of the reproductive organs can also be healed. Practicing will increase your sensitivity to the Qi, and you will soon be able to detect even minute quantities of Qi in its journey throughout your body.

The Second Series

This set is usually performed immediately after the first. If you have already performed the first series, there is no need to redo the warm up exercises. There are three exercises in the Second Series: Cross Hands, Red-Crowned Phoenix Greets the Dawn, and Immortals Guiding the Road. These are performed to strengthen the organs in the Triple Burner area.

The Triple Burner is identified in Chinese medicine as one of the six Yang organs: the gall bladder, stomach, small intestine, large intestine, and bladder being the others. These organs admit, break down, and assimilate food and expel waste. The Triple Burner is conceived of as a system of organs in the central region of the body. This organ system is generally considered to be the lungs, spleen, and kidneys, but sometimes the small intestines and bladder are included as well. So, the Triple Burner does not exist except as a composite of the other organs.

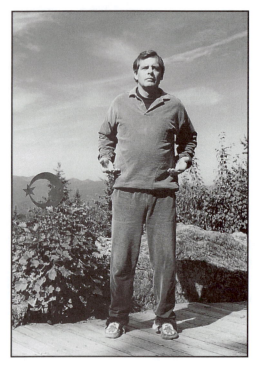

Natural Stance, opening
position: palms up.

THE NATURAL STANCE

All three exercises in this set are performed from the Natural Stance.
This is another stance in which your legs are shoulder width apart,
and your knees are only very slightly bent. Let your arms hang
loosely by your side. Raise your hands until they are waist height,
nearly touching the beltline. Palms should face to the sky. Now
make a reverse circling motion, so that your hands move behind
your body. Let your hands come to rest in the starting position at
the beltline.

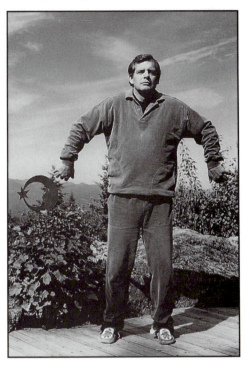

Palms circle behind body and then return to starting position.

CROSS HANDS

From the Natural Stance, bring your hands all the way around behind your body, just as you did to open into the Natural Stance. Rather than returning your hands to the side of your body, cross the wrists at the level of the sternum, with your right hand on the inside. Your right thumb should be just touching the sternum. Your hands should now be back-to-back with your fingers pointing to the underside of your throat. As you open into this position, breathe in. This position is called the Standing Palm.

With your back straight, bend slightly at the heels and stretch your arms out in front of your body, making certain your wrists remain crossed. Try not to let your wrists slip from their positions, which should be as centered against each other as possible.

As you move your arms forward, breathe out. Keep your fingers pointing straight up. Your body is bent slightly at a 70-degree

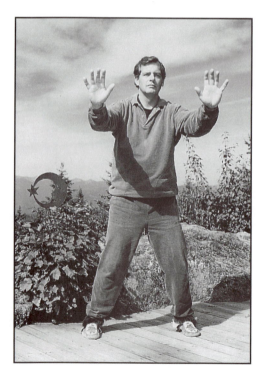

Palms circle in front of body.

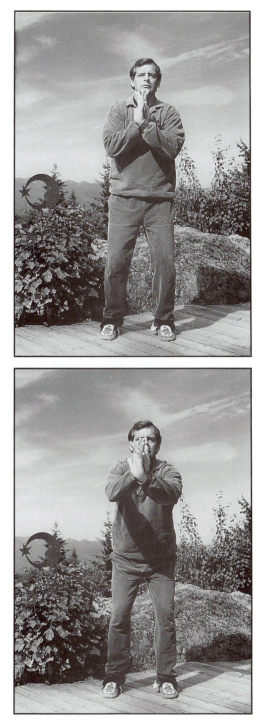

Standing palm position.

Extend arms, bend at waist.

angle at the waist, and your legs should be straight, with your knees in a locked position. Hold this posture for 3 seconds. Now draw your hands back to your chest, breathing in with the movement. Hold for another 3 seconds.

This is one set. Do 10 sets and then return to the Natural Stance, with hands at the hips and palms to the sky. Draw your wrists together again in the Standing Palm position, this time with the left hand on the inside, touching the sternum. Do 10 more sets, remembering to breathe out as you extend your hands, and to breathe in as you retract them.

During the forward motion, the Qi rises from the heels, moves through the calves, knees, hips, trunk, and arms, and finally to your hands, palms, and fingers. When pulling your palms back to your chest, your legs should be slightly bent. Remember to keep your neck and shoulder muscles as relaxed as possible.

In this exercise, the outward motion of the Standing Palm tightens many of the muscles along your back. This, in turn, causes Yang Qi to rise from the feet up through the length of your body. The return motion relaxes the muscles and the Qi flows back down. The pushing and pulling motion massages the blood vessels along the spine. Regular practice encourages the free flow of Qi along the Governing Vessel (chapter 5: page 160). One major benefit from this exercise is that it not only helps prevent future back pain, but it also diminishes existing pain.

RED-CROWNED PHOENIX
GREETS THE DAWN

From the Natural Stance, move your right hand in an arc in front of your body. Make sure your hand does not move more than five or six inches from your body during its travels. On its journey, your palm moves from a face up to a face down position. You should begin to turn it over about halfway along toward the center of your body. It comes to rest about two inches (10 centimeters) directly above the left palm, so that the two palms are aligned over their respective centers at the Laogong point. Let the palms communicate with one another for three seconds.

As you move your hand, breathe in. The whole motion from one side to the other should take exactly as much time as it takes to draw a full, unhurried breath. Then make the return motion, exhal-

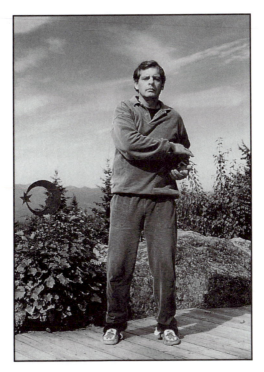

Two palms communicating.

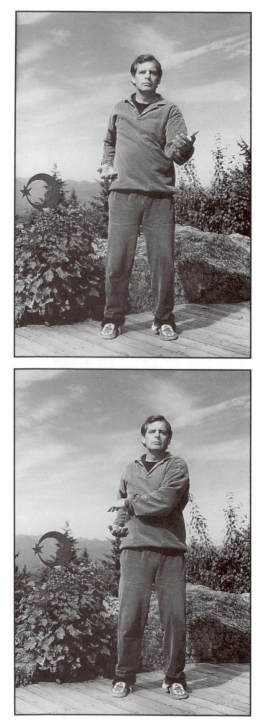

Lower palm remains still,
upper palm returns.

Alternate palm moves into
position.

ing and making the hissing sound as you do. Remember to turn your palm over so that it is face up again.

Next move the left hand, breathing in, and turning it over as before, until it reaches the right palm. After a 3-second pause, move it back again, remembering to exhale and to make the hissing sound. The Red-Crowned Phoenix has now greeted the dawn once. Greet the Dawn 10 times in all.

As your hand moves in front of your body, be aware of the Qi. It will be particularly noticeable when your palms are communicating. Over time, this practice will lead to a heightened awareness of Qi, and it should become an integral part of your study. Heightened awareness of this life force is a key to mastery of this discipline. Special knowledge of this living energy will eventually enable you to recognize it as it moves through your body.

Moving your hand back in front of the body along the Belt Channel (chapter 5: page 165) as you inhale enables you to collect Universal Qi and to store it internally. Regular practice will greatly increase your ability to exchange Qi with the universe.

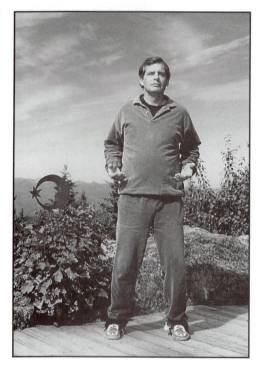

Natural Stance.

IMMORTALS GUIDING THE ROAD

From the Natural Stance, lean forward at the waist, keeping your back and neck straight. Extend your arms, being aware of the internal strength which originates in your feet and calves. This power is amplified in turn by your legs, hips, trunk, and arms. In this exercise, you are attempting to raise the Qi from the abdominal region to the chest level.

Your arms sweep forward in an upward arc. At their lowest level, your arms should remain above your lower abdomen (Lower Burner). At their highest level, they should not rise above the upper chest (Upper Burner).

You do not want to raise the Qi to the level of your head. When your arms reach a comfortable forward position (you do not need to stretch to the point of discomfort) pause for 3 seconds. Then turn your palms over so they are facing the earth. Now retract

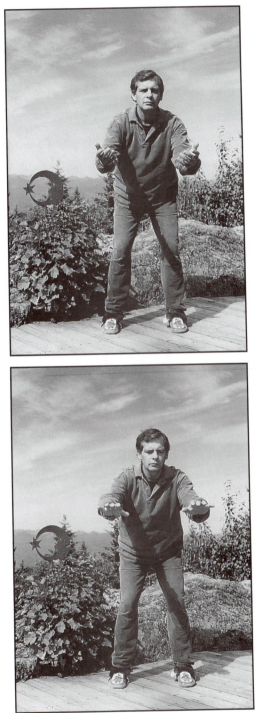

Bend at waist making
scooping motion.

Palms reverse position to
face earthward.

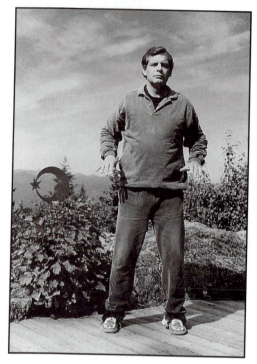

Palms at hips just before
reversing to face skyward.

them, so that you are once again standing in the Natural Stance.
When your palms are close to the body, turn them over again. The
Immortal has Guided the Road once. Guide the Road 10 times.

In this exercise, your legs, hips, back, and arms are exercised
so that the Qi from the body is collected in the palms and fingertips. From here it can be transmitted externally.

The Third Series

This series is comprised of three exercises: Splitting the Mountain, Pulling the Moon from the Bottom of the Lake, and Lifting the Cauldron. The series is usually performed directly after the first two. All three exercises are done from the Wide Stance, a variation of the Natural Stance described below. Make the Natural Stance one step wider than usual. This is the Wide Stance.

If you have already done the warm ups for the first series, there is no need to redo them. This group of exercises promotes the flow of Yang energy up the body through your legs and out into your arms and fingers.

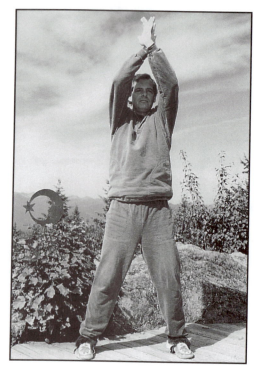

Wide Stance, Standing Palm
position, arms extended
over head.

SPLITTING THE MOUNTAIN
(SPLITTING T'AI SHAN WITH AN AX)

In his book, *T'ai Shan: An Account of the Sacred Eastern Peak of China*,
Dwight Bahu notes that this mountain is wellknown in the East as
holy ground. Historically, it has been sacred ground for at least
2000 years before the Christian era and has served as a stronghold
for the Taoists. Although it is not especially high or difficult to
climb, it is still the journey's end for pilgrims from many countries.
Knowing this history, performing the exercise might be considered
the act of an iconoclast.

Make the Natural Stance one step wider than usual. This is
referred to as the Wide Stance. Your hands should open as they
would in a Natural Stance, hands at belt level, palms facing up.
Now assume the Standing Palm position.

Inhale as you move your hands directly up over your head.
When your hands have reached the zenith, slice the mountain by

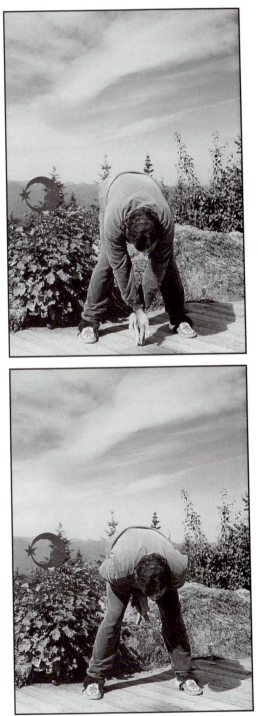

Bend at waist to
"Split the Mountain."

Hands return to solar plexus.

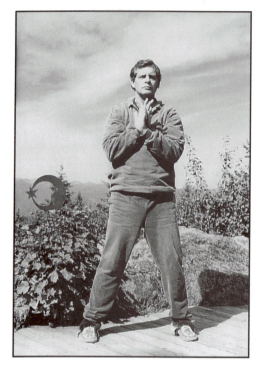

Stand up, fingers beneath chin.

bending forward at the hips, keeping your back straight and head up as much as is comfortable. Bend until your hands are at ground level. Now, without changing your posture, pull your arms up so your hands meet at the solar plexus. Only then do you straighten up, still not bending the spine. Do 10 sets and then resume the Standing Palm position, only this time with your left hand on the inside. Do another 10 sets.

In this exercise, remember to keep your legs straight, your knees locked, your head up, and your neck relaxed and not stiff. This exercise brings the Yang energy up the legs and back. As an added benefit, it strengthens the points in the neck by massaging them.

PULLING THE MOON FROM THE BOTTOM OF THE LAKE

From the Wide Stance, assume the Standing Palm position. Breathing in, swing the arms out to the sides so that the palms of your hands are pushing against some invisible object. Breathing out, bend at the hips, and dip your hands into the lake to retrieve the moon. Imagine the moon as a circular object between your feet at ground level. Keep your head up as much you can and still remain comfortable. Breathing in, bring the moon up to the solar plexus by straightening up at the waist. Move the hands in a circle once more behind the body, and cross the wrists again in front, this time with the left hand closest to the body. Do 10 sets.

As in Splitting the Mountain, remember to keep the knees straight, the head up, and the neck relaxed and not stiff.

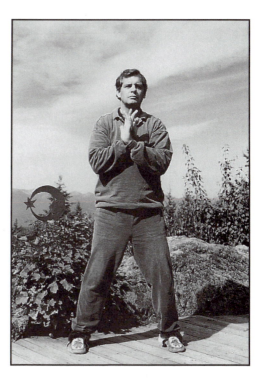

Wide Stance, Standing Palm
position.

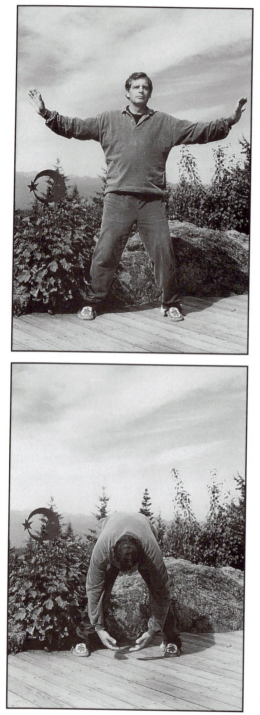

Extend arms out to sides.

Scoop up the Moon.

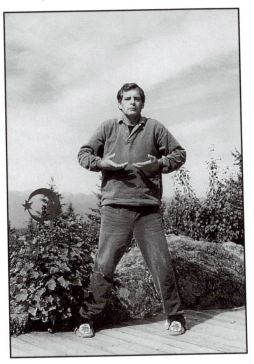

Pull the Moon to solar
plexus level.

Remembering to do this keeps your neck in line with the rest of your spine. As always, breathe in through the nose and out through the mouth. This exercise brings the Yang energy up your legs and back. It strengthens the points in the neck by massaging them. As well, it moves the energy out the arms and into the fingertips.

LIFTING THE CAULDRON
(THE KING LIFTS THE INCENSE POT)

From the Wide Stance, draw both hands inward, palms up, so that your fingertips almost meet at the solar plexus. Breathing in, Lift the Cauldron up to your chest. When your hands reach the upper chest, in one motion turn them over so that your palms face to the sky. Still breathing in and without pausing, extend them over the head so that the palms are to the sky, using some force to do so. Now breathing out, let your arms move outward to the sides of the body. Bend your wrists and let the arms scoop inwardly so that the fingertips nearly meet again at the solar plexus. Do 10 sets.

The legs and back are straight and motionless during this exercise. As a result of the arm and hand movement, the Qi is moved in and out of the body through the fingertips.

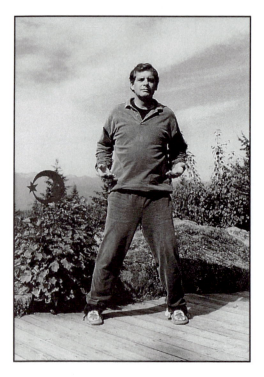

Wide Stance, palms skyward.

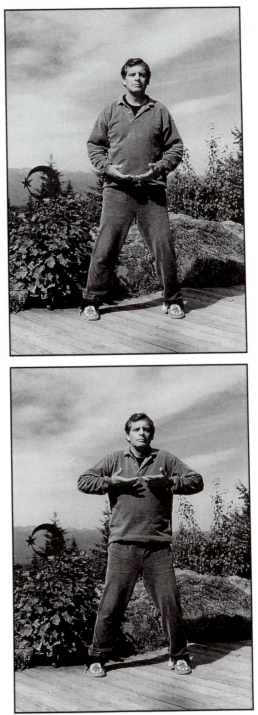

Fingers almost touching at solar plexus.

Lift the cauldron.

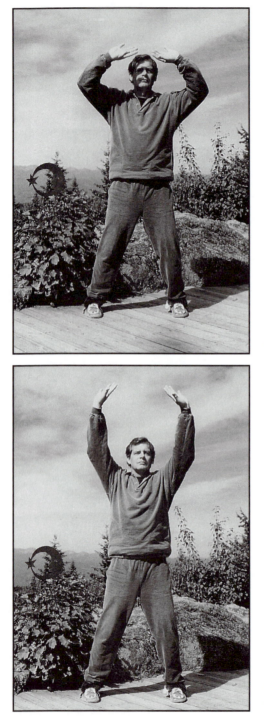

Turn palms over, raise cauldron above head.

Arms return to fingertip position, forming great circle.

The Fourth Series

After the first three series are learned, this final set can
be added. It should be performed immediately after the
first three although, if you do not have enough time, it
can be left until another part of the day. The exercises
enable the practitioner to strengthen the Qi and to
absorb it into the body. These exercises are called
Pulling the Qi and Changing the Qi.

PULLING THE QI

In the Natural Stance, with the knees relaxed, bring both hands in toward the waist so that the two palms face each other directly in front of the Shimen point. This is called Holding the Ball. As has been mentioned, when you feel the energy exchange between your palms, it is said that your hands are in communication. The palms remain in communication for the duration of this exercise even though their relative position changes.

Move the left hand to a 45-degree angle, so that it faces partially skyward. Since the palms are communicating, the right hand should also move to a complementary angle centered over the left palm and face partially earthward. Inhaling through the nose, extend both hands; the right moves up while the left moves down.

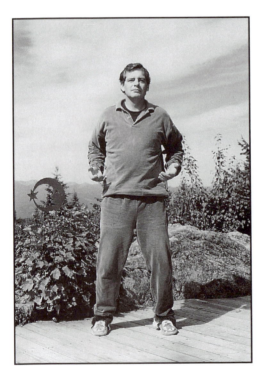

Natural Stance.

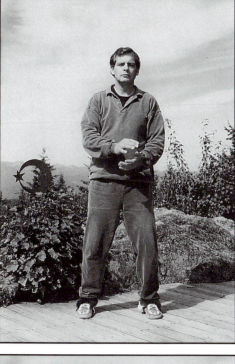

Two palms communicating at
an angle.

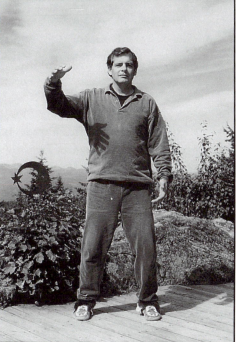

Stretching the Qi.

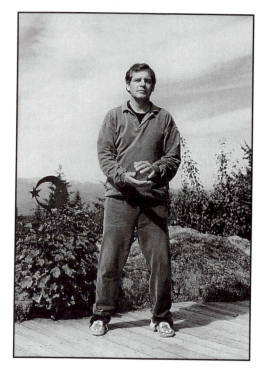

Hands reversed: compressing the Qi.

Take care not to move your arms more than a few inches away from your body. The upper right hand should move to a spot about shoulder height while the lower left hand should move to a spot level with your hip.

It is very important that the Laogong points in the center of the palms are consistently in alignment. When they are stretched to their maximum, exhale and slowly bring the hands toward each other again. A few inches before they actually meet, reverse the angles and the direction of the pull. The left palm is now above. Both hands should move simultaneously to their positions. When the right hand has been in both the lower and upper positions, one cycle has been completed. Do 10 sets.

This exercise stretches the Qi when the palms move apart and compresses it when they move together. The action strengthens and tones the overall quality of Qi in our body as it is emitted from the palms. The exercise is very effective. There are two variations of this exercise known as The Rain, performed by wiggling the fingertips instead of holding them still and The Wind, performed by slightly waving the palms at one another in sequence. These two variations are usually done after Pulling the Qi. You may notice the Qi as interesting tingling sensations in your hands and arms.

CHANGING THE QI

From a Natural Stance, with the knees relaxed, breathe in and circle your hands behind the body so that they meet together in front
of your body in the prayer position. Apply some force when your
palms meet each other. Exhale and stretch both arms out to the
sides of the body with the palms out. When they reach their maximum extent, again apply some force, as if you were pushing
against an invisible object. Breathing naturally, extend your right
arm straight up above your head, as if your palm were holding up
the heavens.

At the same time, the left hand should move to its lowest
extent along the center-of-body line. Just before reaching the far-
thest points above and below the body, you should once more
apply some strength to the stretch so that the muscles in the arms

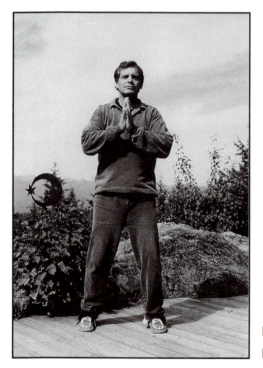

Natural Stance: prayer
position.

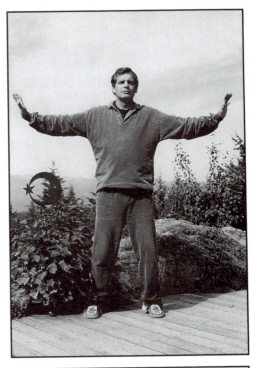

Arms extended to sides.

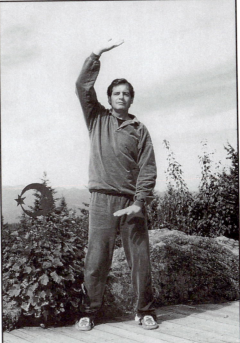

Arms above head.

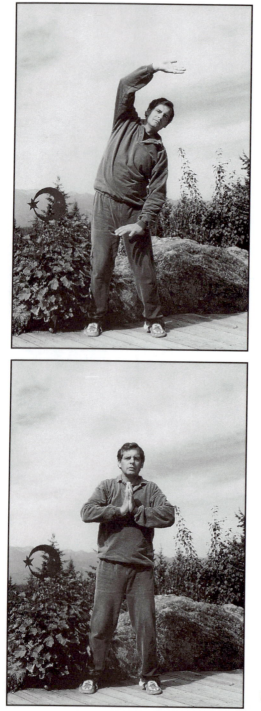

Beginning stretch to side.

Return to prayer position.

and chest are tensed. At this point, imagine your palm holding down the earth.

Breathing out, lean to the left as far as it is comfortable. Then, with your arms still in position, bend the body back to a standing position. Relax your body completely. Breathing in, both arms should be brought into the prayer position at chest level where they are again pressed together with some force.

Continue as before except this time switch arms so the right hand now extends below the body to hold down the earth and the left holds up the heavens. One cycle is completed when the right arm has been in both the top and bottom position. Change the Qi 10 times.

This exercise is excellent for improving the circulation of Qi throughout the body and balancing the Qi on both sides. Bending to the side encourages the maximum amount of Qi to move up the side that is stretched. Changing the Qi also transforms the Qi developed during practice into a form suitable to be stored in your body.

Closing Exercise

This exercise is performed at the end of your daily practice. Its purpose is to consolidate all of your activities and bring a formal ending to the practice. Since it is louder and more vigorous than the other exercises, people with medical conditions, particularly high blood pressure or heart conditions, should do this gently or not at all. After performing all four sets of exercises, finish with a five-minute Horse Stance. Then, if your physical condition permits, do the following exercise.

WILD HORSES RUSHING TO THE BARN

How the title of the exercise came about I'm not certain. Perhaps in China even the wildest horses have always had a barn. More likely, it is a description of the way the Qi is flowing in the body after practice. Spec, the horse I ride, is definitely not wild. But after a day on the trail, he does like to rush home, whether I want him to or not. He knows very well that there are oats waiting for him.

From the Arrow Stance, place your right hand palm down on your right knee. Now place the back of your left hand face up on top of it. Inhale, shifting your weight backward. The palm resting on the knee follows a line up the leg to the hip. Then let your arms swing out to the sides of your body and draw your hands together to make fists at the waist. With your right hand (that rested on your knee) slightly higher than the other, push your fists out and up in

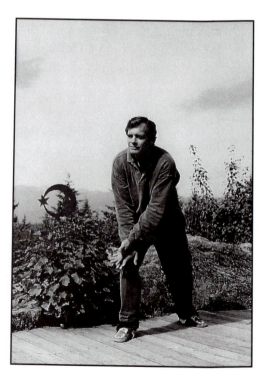

Arrow Stance, hands rest
on knees.

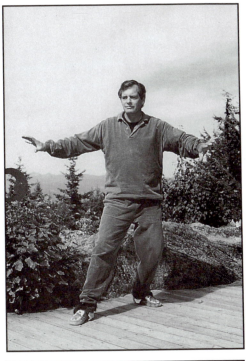

Preparing to make fists.

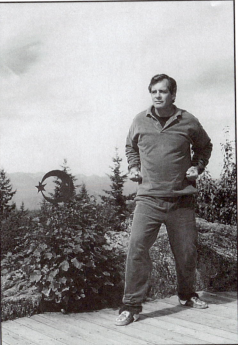

Fists at sides.

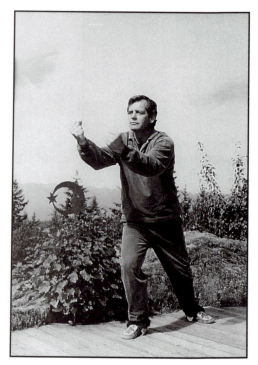

Arms moving upward,
preparing to shout.

a quick motion, shouting HHHEEE, HHHAAA or even HHEEAA as you do. Repeat this seven times and then perform the exercise with the left leg forward.

CHAPTER 3

The Healing Aspects of Qi and Qi Gong

In terms of how practitioners use Qi for healing purposes, three general categories can be presented: Yang or hot Qi, Yin, or cold Qi, and Spiral, or penetrative, Qi. Yang Qi can be used to treat most ailments but Yin Qi is far superior for certain problems, such as twisted necks, sprains, fevers, and so on. It is inadvisable to treat a Yin problem with Yin Qi as this might compound the difficulty. At this level of practice, though, exercises to cultivate cold Qi are not given, so the possibility of emitting cold Qi will not occur. Spiral Qi has a great ability to penetrate living tissues and it can be used to remove difficult blockages in the channels. It is only by learning advanced forms of Qi Gong that you will be able to emit either Spiral or cold Qi. Spiral Qi, by the way, can be emitted to a distance of about 16 feet.

One skill advanced practitioners often develop is the ability to see auras around areas of affliction, such as in an organ, a muscle, or other tissue. This light reflects the colors associated with the particular affliction. Once this extrasensory skill is developed, practitioners are able to use auras as diagnostic tools. For example, depending on the severity or type of problem, a green, light blue, or white light can be seen around the stomach areas of people with chronic indigestion. If the light is green, a practitioner may be able to tell whether or not it is just indigestion or if the problem is an actual inflammation. If the practitioner continues to emit Qi and the color does not change, then the patient has an ulcer. If, on the other hand, the color changes quickly, then it is not a serious problem. Ulcers and other major problems can be healed using Qi Gong techniques but to do so requires prolonged treatment.

Qi gates are acupuncture points which have special significance in the channels. As the name implies, the gates are points which permit the entry or exit of large volumes of Qi. The opening of these Qi gates by a Master is an important step if students wish to be able to develop their full capacity to work with others. The opening of these gates is only meaningful after diligent practice. It is important to note that if students do not practice, gates which have been opened will close by themselves. Opening Qi gates, though, is not a requirement for personal health, and as I have already mentioned, the technique is most useful to enhance your work with others.

If you notice a cold area in the body, particularly around the soles of the feet, during practice, or when treating others, it is an indication that the Yin Qi is starting to move. This is a good sign because it means that it is now easier for hot Qi to move into the afflicted area. Noticing these kinds of subtle changes suggests that you are developing your ability to distinguish among the different forms of Qi, and that you are also able to actually move it through the body.

APPLICATIONS FOR SPECIFIC AILMENTS

While Qi Gong can be used to treat practically any human affliction, it is most commonly used to treat or prevent the following common diseases.

- Respiratory ailments, such as the flu, colds, asthma, tracheitis (inflammation of the trachea), bronchitis, pulmonary emphysema.

- Digestive ailments, such as prolapsed stomach, ulcers, chronic hepatitis, cholecystitis (gall bladder inflammation), gall stones, indigestion, constipation, and diarrhea. While just a few treatments will give good results for some of these problems, a disease as severe as a prolapsed stomach will take much more work.

- Circulatory system dysfunction, such as high blood pressure, rheumatic heart disease, arrhythmia (irregular heart beat), hypertension (patients can reduce their level of tension by a significant degree after just a few treatments), coronary thrombosis (hardening of the arteries).

- Urinary and reproductive system concerns with kidneys, impotence, elimination of wastes, dysmenorrhoea (difficult or painful menstruation), prolapsed uterus.

- Nervous system breakdowns which cause general weakness, such as neurasthenia (weak nerves), pains in the ribs or back, numbness of nerves, insomnia, headaches, migraine, sciatic pains (pains of the hip or sciatic nerve), and some kidney complaints.

- Arthritis, rheumatism, general pains in shoulders, knees, lower back, neck twists (these can often be healed overnight), wrist pains, chilblains (an inflammatory swelling of the hands or feet due to excessive exposure to cold).

- Eyes, ears, nose, and throat problems, such as false short-sightedness, some hearing difficulties, rhinitis (inflammation of the nose), pharyngitis (inflammation of the pharynx), general inflammations of ears, nose, and throat.

- This type of Qi Gong is not especially effective with mental conditions. Psychotics and schizophrenics should not practice this form themselves. It can be helpful, though, for those with only a mild condition.

METHODOLOGY

Most people cannot generate enough Qi by themselves to over-come serious diseases. One of the functions of a Qi Gong practi-tioner is to turn on the internal "Qi switch" in another person. Once the Qi is flowing freely through this person, there is an opportuni-ty to begin treatment. The practitioner initiates this assistance in the following way.

Ask the patient to lie quietly on a standard treatment table. Make certain that this person is lying prone without crossing either arms or legs. Limbs crossed, such as one leg over the other or arms folded over the chest indicates an attitude of psychologi-cal resistance. The physical act of uncrossing these limbs will help your subject to relax. It is also helpful to explain why you are doing this.

Stand over the patient from the side, flutter your fingers and wave your hands, palm down, in a graceful motion up and down the body but over the Triple Burner area in particular. By making these motions, you are stimulating the Qi in the patient's body. The fluttering motion of your fingers enables you to emit Qi. The up-and-down motion of your palms draws the patient's Qi to the sur-face. At the same time, it pushes your own Qi downward to the body's surface. Here, both forces meet. During the whole process your hands never need to come closer than a few inches from the other person. As with much of this practice, physical contact is not necessary.

After five minutes of "Butterfly Hands," as I call this motion, begin moving both hands together down the length of the patient's body from the top of the cranium to as far as you can reach down the legs. The exact distance of your hands above your patient's body will be anywhere from six inches to two feet depending on the height of the treatment table. The most impor-tant thing is to stay relaxed and comfortable. The hand motions balance the Qi in the body, and begin to move it naturally through the channels. Do this for another five minutes or until you notice that the patient is completely relaxed. If a second practitioner is

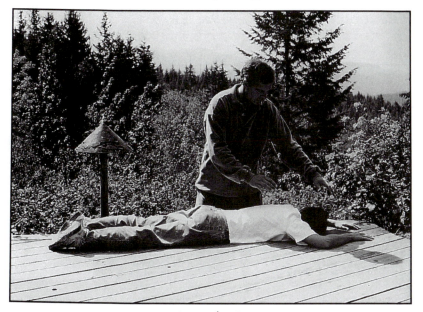

Moving the Qi.

present, have this person pull (or draw) the Qi from the sole of the patient's foot.

During this stage, be aware of how your hands feel as they pass over certain parts of the body. If they feel cool or cold, there is a deficiency of Yang Qi and an excess of Yin Qi. If you feel excessive heat, the reverse is true. Both conditions indicate a problem. As I have said elsewhere in the text, even if you cannot "see" the Qi or aura, you still may be able to feel it. This sense, when fully developed, is a very useful diagnostic tool. If at first you cannot notice anything unusual, ask what the problem might be. Table 4 on page 102 indicates the types of sensations you will be able to feel with your hands. Eventually you may even be able to see them. Notice how the range of possible sensations follows a pattern of opposites.

The application of Qi affects each of us in different ways, but there are certain very obvious similarities common to everyone. These can be described as being akin to the influences of hypnotism. Most notable of these are the progressive relaxation of the body, the regulation of the breathing, and eventually the induction of a trancelike state. The depth of this trance depends on the qual-

Table 4 : Characteristics of Qi in the Human Body.

SENSATION	INTERPRETATION
Hot	There is an excess of Qi.
Cold	There is a deficiency of Qi.
Attracting	The patient's Qi complements and welcomes your own.
Repelling	The patient's Qi rejects your own.
Steady	The flow of Qi is dependable.
Irregular	Qi moves through the body as if it must circumnavigate obstacles.
Thick	There is a substantial, generous quality about the Qi.
Thin	Qi is distributed over too great a volume for its substance.
Hollow	The Qi has a strong outer appearance but is without any real force.
Fast	The Qi is racing through the body, generating excess heat.
Slow	The patient's energy levels are not at their peak.
Strong	The Qi is powerful and enduring.
Weak	The Qi is frail and tenuous.
Rigid	There is an inflexible quality about the Qi.
Loose	The Qi moves without apparent direction.

ities of both patient and practitioner. After you have stimulated and regulated the Qi and searched for abnormalities, you can begin to emit Qi directly over the region, organ or tissue in question. This method is referred to as treating by direct radiation. There are variations of this method. One commonly used technique is to amplify the emission of Qi by focusing both hands, one on top of the other, over the part of the body to be treated. (See illustration below.)

You can also use tools to direct Qi. Sandalwood fans emit a wonderful fragrance and are used to heal lung infections and other respiratory problems. The practitioner unfolds the fan, and waves it in front of the patient's nostrils, emitting Qi all the while. The fragrance, together with all its healing properties, is carried by the Qi deep into the body tissues. Another significant technique which relies on tools is that of moxibustion, a method of inducing heat into a point or region by the external application of chemically created heat. Moxa, the "wool" used as a heat source, is made from the dried leaves of the mugwort plant (artemisia vulgaris). This plant has been used in China for at least two thousand years. It is knead-

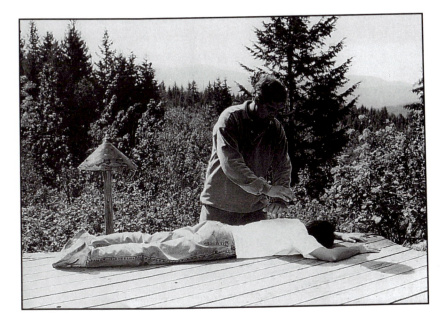

Direct radiation using two hands.

ed into cones of various sizes and shapes, and when it burns, it has the property of dispelling unhealthy Qi. When directed by the practitioner's Qi, the heat can be very effective in certain situations such as asthma, chronic indigestion, painful conditions of the joints, and even in cases of toxic insect bites. Moxa is often used in conjunction with ginger, salt, garlic or applied in stick form.

The most common method of treating with Qi is to emit it from either the palms or the fingertips. Your choice will depend on the purpose at hand. Qi can also be emitted from the center of the fore-head, from the solar plexus, and from the feet as well. For obvious reasons, using these parts of the anatomy in your daily routine is not always practical. For general practice, palms or fingertips will do. If you need to remove a blockage in a channel, you would prob-ably use your index finger, closing the others. Closing the rest of the fingers (and this simply means bending them until they are folded over) blocks the flow of Qi in them. This makes more Qi available to flow from your index finger and also gives you greater control by allowing you to direct the Qi at specific points.

In a situation where you are treating an organ, such as a lung, you would likely use your palms. Since the surface of the palms is greater than in a finger, you will emit Qi over a wide area. Spend no more than ten minutes, at most, working with someone during the initial stages of your practice. Your body requires time to develop skill in collecting Qi as well as in emitting it. There is no point in depleting your own vital energies in your efforts to heal. Later, after a year or two of practicing Shaolin Nei Jin Qi Gong, you will be able to treat patients for an hour or two without difficulty. Advanced practitioners can treat patients all day without adverse effects.

Two of the central diagnostic problems occur in trying to decide how and where to apply Qi. Resolving these difficulties involves identifying which channel requires treatment, the location of its acupuncture points and the selection of the most appropriate points to treat. This is why a thorough knowledge of the basic prin-ciples of acupuncture is invaluable.

When you are finished treatment, ask the patient to lie com-fortably for several minutes. Then ask the person to sit up on the table. Gently massage the neck, shoulders, and back using a Qi

Gong massage. This pushes the Qi into the body and helps prevent dizziness and disorientation. The method involves moving your hands in a circular motion on, or sometimes just above, the surface of the patient's body. Move your hands in this manner 20 times, first in a clockwise and then in the opposite direction an equal number of times. A Qi Gong massage is always very light, so that there is almost no pressure at all. It is very common for the patient to feel sleepy during this massage. This is another reason you ask patients to sit up before massaging.

While results of Qi Gong treatment are not always immediate, once Qi is imparted to the patient, it remains in that body's tissues and acts to reinforce existing Qi. It will continue to work that evening, for the next day, and even longer in some cases.

Over time the patient can often learn to move the Qi alone. Once the patient can sense the Qi and understand the related principles, there is every reason to expect that he or she will assume some of the responsibility for effecting a cure. Common sense dictates that if the patient is actively involved as an enthusiastic partner in the healing process, the chances of a cure will be greatly enhanced. This is certainly true in other fields such as education or psychology and the result of failing to involve the patient are evidenced by the time-honored adage, "You can lead a horse to water but you can't make it drink." Put another way, if you can gain the confidence and the cooperation of the patient, you will have a greatly improved session.

ANTON MESMER'S DISCOVERY OF QI

One interesting historical case is that of Anton Mesmer who pioneered "hypnotic" techniques in 18th-century Europe (circa. 1765). I have placed the word hypnotic in quotes because it is clear from the descriptions of his methods that Mesmer did not use the same type of hypnosis we are familiar with today. He used methods remarkably similar to our own in Qi Gong. In fact, his technique was nicknamed *animal magnetism* and was performed by repeatedly passing the hands over the body. This sounds very much like the first two stages of awakening and moving the Qi in our own practice.

Mesmer's methods contained a substantial proportion of theatricality, and it is difficult to ascertain the direct causes for his cures (of which there were a remarkable number). The following quotation from the text *Medical and Dental Hypnosis and Its Clinical Applications* by John Hartland illustrates Mesmer's predisposition toward showmanship.

> *Mesmer, the great magnetizer, now appeared, wearing a silken robe of a pale lilac color, and holding in his hand a long iron wand. He passed slowly through the ranks, fixing his eye upon the patients, passing his hand over their body or touching them with his iron wand. Many patients were unable to notice much result and declared that they could feel absolutely nothing. But some of the patients coughed, spat and felt as if insects were running all over their skin. Finally some, especially young women, would fall down and go into convulsions.*[1]

After several sessions, many people declared themselves healed. There is no doubt in my own mind that Mesmer's use of the Qi was partly responsible for his "miracles." In fact, it also seems probable that Mesmer had direct instruction in this art. Hartland describes Mesmer's beliefs about his own healing techniques in the following way.

> *He supposed the human body to be influenced by the planets through the instrumentality of an invisible magnetic fluid. He called this fluid, which had many properties resembling those of a magnet, the fluid of animal magnetism. He considered disease to be caused by an inharmonious distribution of this fluid in the patient's body. Consequently, in making his "passes" a*

---

1. John Hartland, *Medical & Dental Hypnosis & Its Clinical Applications,* 2nd ed. (London: Baillière Tindall, 1982), p. 5.

few inches from the body-surface, Mesmer believed that invisible magnetic fluid flowed out of his finger-tips into the patient's body, achieving the necessary redistribution and restoring the balance. Once this had been effected, the patient regained his health.[2]

Mesmer was remarkably successful in healing people who had been declared incurable by the medical establishment. Unfortunately for Mesmer, the medical establishment of the day issued a decree outlawing the practice, thereby retarding its study for many generations. Interestingly, two members of the investigation committee, who concluded fraud on the part of Mesmer, were Benjamin Franklin, scientist and founding father of the United States, and Dr. Guillotine, who invented the device used to execute the aristocracy during the French Revolution.

In our own century, the practice of hypnosis, until recently at least, has been treated in much the same way. Ironically, Mesmer's natural allies, the hypnotists, today often completely disregard the techniques of "animal magnetism" as being unfounded in science and endorse only their own psychological approaches. What should be understood is that there are two distinct methods involved, those of modern psychology and those of Traditional Chinese Medicine. Each of these has its own procedures and theory and each is perfectly viable within its own sphere of influence.

To underscore the importance of this last point, I am including another reference to Mesmerism and its beneficial effects in medical practice. James Esdaile, M.D., wrote about his experiences with Mesmerism in his book *Hypnosis in Medicine and Surgery*. Originally titled *Mesmerism in India*, it was first published in 1850. This text offers a wealth of details about the practical medical applications of Qi (through Mesmerism in this case) in a situation which did not offer the conveniences of modern surgical practice. It is curious to note that the title of the 1957 edition has been changed from the original, replacing the word Mesmerism with

---

2. Hartland, *Medical & Dental Hypnosis & Its Clinical Applications*, p. 5.

Hypnosis. This change probably reflects the legal and social climate of the day. At any rate, Dr. Esdaile's notes clearly indicate that he used "animal magnetism" to effect his results, and he did not employ the psychological approaches of modern hypnosis.

While the results of his work were remarkable, Esdaile comments that Mesmer's theatricality brought about his own downfall. He states in a rather dramatic fashion:

> But Nature, like an over-loaded camel, turned upon her driver, and threw him and his paraphernalia of magnetic platforms, conducting-rods and ropes, pianos, magnetized trees and buckets, into the dirt; and truth retired in disgust to the bottom of her well, there to dwell till more honest men should draw her forth again to surprise and benefit the world.[3]

Notwithstanding his criticism, Esdaile's text really is a testament to the effectiveness of Mesmerism, and there is no question in his mind that it was a very real and beneficial force. Who better to know than a practicing medical doctor? Today accepting invisible vital forces is much easier than in the doctor's day. Our understanding of particle physics is now far in advance of the physical science of that age. We do not question the idea that all things above a temperature of absolute zero exist in a state of motion and that objects only appear to be solid. Electron microscopes, which enable us to magnify matter a million times, have left us with no doubt that in its rudimentary forms, matter is anything but solid. As a result of the transmission of the wisdom teachings from the East to this hemisphere, the Western world has acquired a philosophical background with sufficient depth to help us interpret these kinds of discoveries.

We also have photographic techniques mentioned earlier (chapter 1, page 12) that can actually capture an image of the aura surrounding living tissues on film. This quality of empirical evidence has left even the most jaded cynics with little option but to

---

3. James Esdaile, *Hypnosis in Medicine and Surgery* (New York: Julian Press, 1957), p. 54.

accept the notion that living tissues radiate energy. If this is not enough, we also have biofeedback devices that enable us to track the flow of bioelectrical energy in the body. As a result of these advances we are in a far better position to study Qi (prana) and its associated phenomena than we were a hundred years ago.

Thanks to our benefactors from the East, we now can identify many subtle facts about Qi. We know, for example, that it moves through the body and throughout the universe in the form of a wave, and not in a straight line. This fact has been applied in the martial arts from the earliest of times. The principle is used to amplify strength, to heighten agility, to pinpoint weaknesses and strengths and for many other purposes. We only have to make a brief visit to a martial arts studio or a Qi Gong clinic to see for ourselves some of the many applications of Qi.

THE MOVEMENT OF QI THROUGH MATTER

As I have suggested indirectly, the study of nature reveals that one of the characteristics living things exhibit is this tendency to spiral movement. It appears in the form of growth, in the pattern of leaves on a stem or branches on a tree trunk, in the designs on shells, in the organization of seeds on a flower head and in an unlimited number of other examples. Physical forms in general, whether or not they are alive, reflect the movement of Universal Qi through matter. Watch the formation of waves as they rise, crest, and fall or the examples left by wind on the desert sands. Study the twisted curves on the horns of Bighorn sheep, the petals of flowers, the shape of galaxies, or the scale patterns on fish. All these things reflect the constant movement of Qi through both animate and inanimate matter. You can further explore this profound mystery in a valuable book written by Theodore Andrea Cook, first published in 1914. It is appropriately titled, *The Curves of Life*.

Accomplishing the free flow of Qi in your body requires eliminating any blockages in the channels of your body. When this objective has been reached, the Qi can once again flow naturally. If the Qi is not moving properly certain parts of your body will be deprived of vital nutrition, weaken as a result, and eventually begin to atrophy. Your primary purpose in this work is to first achieve this goal within your own body. The work of the accomplished practitioner, on the other hand, is to abolish these blockages in others.

BENDING-FINGER METHOD FOR CURING AILMENTS

Since there are a great number of Qi gates in the hands, it stands to reason that exercising them in specific ways will promote the flow of Qi down their associated channels. Since each of the fingers is associated with an internal organ or group of organs, these exercises are beneficial for the health of the entire body. The general associations of fingers with the rest of the body are indicated in Table 5.

By exercising your fingers using the special techniques of Shaolin Nei Jin Qi Gong, you will promote the development of Qi and its vital flow in your body. This flow will adjust and regulate the functioning of the organs, and the Bending-Finger Method will

Table 5: The Fingers and their Anatomical Relationships.

FINGER	ORGAN	AREA OF BODY	TYPE
Thumb	Lung	Head	Yin
Index	Large Intestine	Collarbone to Diaphragm	Yang
Little (top)	Small Intestine	Shimen* to Feet	Yang
Little (bottom)	Heart	Shimen to Feet	Yin
Middle	Pericardium	Diaphragm to Navel	Yin
Ring	Triple Burner	Navel to Shimen	Yang

* Shimen point, Ren No. 5, also discussed on pages 23, 24, and 163.

attract, guide, and properly redistribute your vital body energy. Another interesting feature of this exercise is that it will reduce the overall amount of time you must spend with the other Qi Gong exercises to achieve the results you desire. Practicing will also enable you to emit Qi through your fingers, the first requirement of anyone who wishes to use Qi for healing. When you master this, you will also be able to promote and regulate the flow of Qi in others.

Bending-finger exercises are also used to treat a number of illnesses. Special sequences of bending fingers are used for specific purposes such as to relieve insomnia, strengthen the immune system or to remove headaches.

A TREATMENT OF DISEASES AND COMMON AILMENTS

These exercises are generally initiated and closed with a five-minute Horse Stance. Each set of finger bends is held for 50 seconds. Then, during the next 7-10 second period, you can raise your fingers to their original resting position and lower the next set. Finger-bending sequences which have been found effective for various ailments follow.

INSOMNIA
- Bend both little fingers simultaneously a total of 11 times;
- Bend the index fingers twice.

HEADACHES
- Bend the thumbs twice, remembering to stretch them outward;
- Bend the little fingers twice;
- Bend the thumbs together with the little fingers 11 times.

LIVER
- Treat liver problems including the early stages of liver cancer in this way:

- Bend the middle and ring fingers together a total of nine times.

MENTAL DISEASES CAUSED BY
THE SPLITTING OF THE NERVE TISSUES

- Bend the thumbs once and return;
- Raise the index fingers slightly above the others (half an inch) then immediately lower. This is one set;
- Do six sets.

HYPERTENSION

- Bend the ring and little fingers once (bend your fingers only where they meet the hand);
- Stretch and bend the thumbs down for five seconds; then bend them half an inch back up and back down again for 45 seconds;
- Bend the ring and little fingers together again, six times in all.

HEART AILMENTS

- Bend the little fingers once;
- Bend the middle fingers once;
- Hold all fingers outstretched for 10 seconds;
- Bend the little fingers once;
- Bend the middle fingers once;
- Stop for five or 10 seconds;
- The above sequence represents one set;
- Do 11 sets in all.

HOT ASTHMA

This problem is always caused by a fever, a flu, or by the beginnings of pneumonia. One of its symptoms is the frequent expelling of thick mucus.

- Bend the thumb and middle fingers so that the tips of these fingers will be very close to one another but do not touch;

- Do this 9 times;
- Bend the little fingers twice.

COLD ASTHMA
- Symptoms are running noses with clear mucus, colds, shivering, and feeling chilly;
- Bend the thumbs and ring fingers so that they are close to but not touching one another;
- Bend these nine times;
- Bend the middle fingers three times.

STOMACH PROBLEMS
- Bend the middle fingers once;
- Bend the ring fingers once;
- Do 11 sets.

For the Prevention of Cancer

Although this disease is difficult to treat, regardless of the medical system used, the patient can help prevent cancer by performing this set of Bending-Finger exercises. Since this is such an insidious disease, I will describe the exercise in some detail.

During the entire exercise, use natural breathing. Begin with a five minute Horse Stance. While still in the Horse Stance, bend the little fingers of both hands simultaneously for 50 seconds. Next, bend the middle fingers for 50 seconds, and then the thumbs for the same length of time. When bending thumbs, remember to turn them out and stretch them somewhat. Allow a 10-second interval while changing fingers.

Bend the thumb and ring finger of the right hand and move them slowly across the front of the body to the Shaohai point, Heart (H) channel No. 3 (chapter 5: page 140), located below the left elbow of the arm outstretched in the Horse Stance. Move the right hand far enough so your wrist is beneath the Shaohai point and leave it there for three seconds. Now extend this arm as far as possible away from your body (toward the opposite wall) after contact with the Shaohai point.

Pause for the count of three before bringing the arm slowly back into position, and then move the left wrist under the Shaohai point on the right arm. Hold it there for three seconds and again reach for the far wall. Return your arm to its normal position in the Horse Stance. Repeat the sequence nine times in all and then close by holding the Horse Stance for five more minutes.

We bend the little and middle fingers in the beginning because they are connected with the heart and the pericardium respectively. The heart, as you know, is primarily responsible for circulating the blood in the body. The thumb is connected with the lungs, which are related to the function of breathing and oxygenation of the blood. The act of breathing, the substance of air, and the vital energy Qi are three interrelated, but separate factors.

The channels associated with the little and middle fingers cause the unhealthy Qi to rush to the surface of the skin. Once there, we can begin to move this Qi out of the body. The right to left sequence of moving the hands to the Shaohai points injects healthy Qi into the Yin channels. Pulling the arms slowly back into the Horse Stance posture pulls the unhealthy energy into the Yang channels. The in-out motion promotes the circulation of the vital energy and eventually drives the unhealthy energy right out of the body.

According to our practice, cancer is caused because the free flow of Qi has been blocked in its course through the channels. The Qi is then deposited in certain areas and over time it becomes malignant. If you suspect yourself of falling ill to cancer at some point in the future, practice this exercise once a day. For others, practicing once a week will substantially reduce your chances of contracting this disease.

Note that cold sensations felt during this exercise indicate that you are pulling cold and stagnant Qi out of the body. Watching a Master work on someone with cancer reveals the truly sinister nature of this disease. The experience has been likened to having an unusually nasty substance attaching itself to you and having to work very hard to remove it.

For Problems of the Liver & Gallbladder

This area, located below the ribs on the right side of the body, may sometimes feel swollen or expanded. According to Traditional Chinese Medicine, emotions can be stored here, and if they are not dispelled, they can cause discomfort, even though there are not any actual physiological disorders. Eventually, the accumulation of stagnant energy here may affect the workings of the organs them-selves.

Massaging and emitting Qi into the area, and into the knee and leg, will help to start the Qi stored in the area to flow through the body and out the foot. You can also massage the Yanglingquan Gallbladder (G.B.) No. 34 (chapter 5: page 154) and the Dannang point G.B. "New Point" (chapter 5: page 154) just below it for gall bladder problems. (The term "New Point," once called "Extraordi-nary Point," refers to an acupuncture point not included on the original channels. As a result, New Points are not associated with numbers.)

You may also want to use the following exercise. Starting with the Horse Stance, dig your toes deeply into the rug. Bend both your middle and ring fingers of both hands at the same time. Hold this posture for 15 minutes. Return your fingers to the normal out-stretched position, make a hollow Qi Gong fist and close. This tech-nique is referred to as "Removing the Liver Qi" and it is recom-mended to those who suffer from chronic depression or fits of anger.

Another method to relieve liver and gallbladder problems involves lifting the toes of your right foot slightly off the ground but keeping your heel firmly rooted. Use both arms by placing them over the top of your right leg at waist level. With your fingers extended, and without actually touching your leg, push the unhealthy energy down the leg and out through the toes. A varia-tion of this exercise is performed in the following way. Place your right foot on the root of a fir tree and proceed in the same way as in the preceding exercise.

CHAPTER 4

Meditations

The next few pages describe a number of useful meditations and postures. They are, for the most part, directly associated with Qi Gong traditions. All of them are very interesting and will yield promising results to dedicated practitioners. There are people who believe that in the final analysis it matters very little what you meditate on, or which posture you assume when you practice. I do not agree. Many of these meditations or variations of them are hundreds of years old. Each was designed to achieve a specific purpose. Some align specific organs in the body in a unique way. It stands to reason, then, that correct posture is critical in attaining the intended result.

In some respects, understanding the theory behind Qi Gong postures is as important as perfecting the practice itself. The more you learn about the ideas behind the movements, postures, and associations with the natural world, the more advanced your practice will become. If you understand the underlying relationships between the human body and the exercises themselves, you will also be in a stronger position to help others. This is true for the meditations as well as for the actual exercises. If your goal is simply to strengthen your own life energy, or to develop personal psychic abilities, then correct practice alone, without a great deal of attention to the supporting theory, will probably be adequate. There is no doubt, though, that the more we know about our subject, the greater the possibility we have of mastering it in all of its intricacies.

If your aim is to work as a Qi Gong practitioner in a healing clinic, then theory, particularly the ideas in Traditional Chinese Medicine, become vitally important. Above all, there is no substitute for meditation itself, whether you stand or sit. Meditation of almost any sort is preferable to no meditation at all. Use the time to commune with your body, your soul, with the animate and inanimate worlds around you and, if you are very fortunate, with your Creator and the Hierarchy of Beings which populate the universe.

A substantial body of literature on the practice of meditation already exists, and gleanings from this literature indicate that above all, it is through meditation that we secure guidance. Since each of us has the distinction of occupying a unique position on the evolutionary totem pole, meditation naturally is an intensely personal matter. This means that answers to our questions develop in response to our own requirements and abilities. Knowing who we are and why we meditate are two steps we can all take to help ensure practical results of definite spiritual value. By this I mean that it is important to have both a clear vision of our relationship to others and to have specified exactly what it is we hope to achieve in our meditation.

The following meditations can be divided into two general categories. Some deal strictly with the inner processes common to all human beings. Others rely on the interplay between ourselves and the great forces of nature. Most of the meditations fall into this last classification. The distinction is important because in a very basic way these meditations reflect Qi Gong's affinity to the natural world. In a very real sense, this practice is a form of alchemy. By this I mean that practitioners are forever seeking to capture, transform, and make use of the sublime essences found in the world around us.

It is here in the dramatic interaction between the Qi Gong practitioner and the vast, unfathomable forces at play in the universe that we have the clearest sense of the real meaning of Qi Gong and the magic it performs. In the final analysis, we seek to transform the base energies of our bodies into those of a higher, more noble quality. As a result of our efforts, we transform ourselves.

By means of the subtle, ancient forces of Qi Gong, we begin to change. Through study and practice we add depth to our personalities. We rebuild our physical bodies, and we strengthen our characters. The process is gradual, so our transformation is not obvious to others. Without precautions we might even overlook the transformation ourselves. Our special senses develop slowly without being forced. This means that given certain conditions, we have ample opportunity to watch ourselves, to note the manner of our development, and above all to effortlessly integrate our new abilities and characteristics into the regimen of our daily lives.

The Crown

The Qi gate at the crown of the head on the Governing Vessel is known as the Baihui point No. 20 (chapter 4: page 160). It is very important, and is known in Indian metaphysics as the "Crown chakra." When it opens, you will have achieved a fundamental breakthrough in this discipline. If you are seated, meditating, in a darkened room, an opening is indicated by a pillar of gold, white, or purple light which radiates forth through the Baihui point to the ceiling and beyond.

When heaven and earth are united through the illumination of the channels (as evidenced by the awakening of the crown chakra) it is possible to absorb universal Qi and emit it simultaneously.

Gathering the Essence of the Morning Sun

Gathering Essence Qi from the Sun is possible by practicing the Horse Stance, in a very low attitude, when the sun rises. Hold the stance for the first 15 minutes before the sun rises and for 15 minutes after it rises. Being greedy and watching the sun for a longer period can irritate your eyes.

Bend your knees at least three inches over your toes. In fact, for this exercise, the greater the bend in your knees, the more you can absorb the Qi. As you will discover, holding a posture with your knees bent more than three inches past your toes is not easily accomplished.

Fix your eyes on the sun, which appears as a soft, flaming red orb. At this time of the day it is harmless. Later in the morning, it loses its benign quality and becomes the smaller intense orb we typically recall. Just at dawn, though, the sun is beautiful and can induce a sense of divinity.

Although the sun appears red at first, these colors will change as you watch it. This exercise helps develop a form of x-ray vision. When you are finished, massage the Sizhukong acupuncture point,

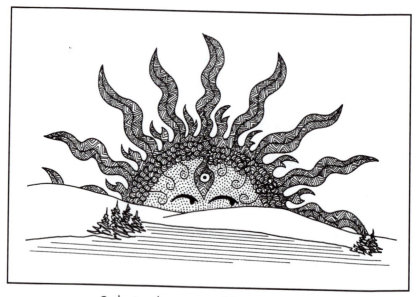

Gathering the essence of the morning sun.

Sanjiao (T.B.) No. 23 (chapter 5: page 150), at the corner of your eyebrows 20 times clockwise and 20 times counterclockwise.

This exercise helps you assimilate certain universal qualities: in essence, you become one with all. When you are finished, do the closing exercise to the Horse Stance. Be sure to dress warmly. If you experience any discomfort from watching the sun, stop at once.

The Life Gate

If the sun rises too high in the sky, the Gathering the Essence of the Morning Sun exercise cannot be carried out. Instead, turn around and let the sun shine on the kidney region. In this way, you can absorb Qi though the Mingmen point, Governing Vessel No. 4 (chapter 5: page 160) on your lower back and replenish your vital energies.

This exercise raises the level of Yang Qi in your body. Rub your hands over the kidneys clockwise and counterclockwise, 40 times each way, to absorb the essence of the sun. The Mingmen point is found on a plane about an inch and a half below the navel on the backside of the body and is known as the "Life Gate."

Performing these exercises at different times during the day will result in different effects. For example, if you were to perform the Life Gate exercise in the evening, the quality of Universal Qi absorbed into your body would be very different from that gained in the early morning. The setting sun has distinct properties, and while it is beautiful in its own right, it has reached the end of its daily cycle. At this time its energies will affect your emotions differently and less favorably than in the morning.

Rabbit Salutes the Goddess of Mercy
(Gathering Energy from the Moon)

This exercise, which involves gathering energy from the moon, is called Rabbit Salutes the Goddess of Mercy. It is performed for each of the three days before, during, and for each of the three days after

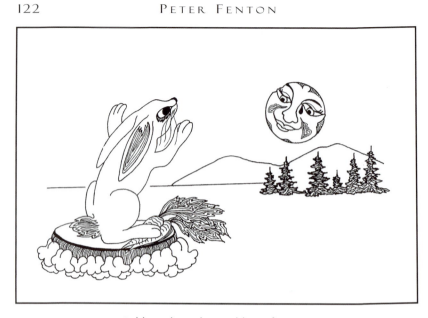

Rabbit salutes the Goddess of Mercy.

the full moon, making a total of seven full days. Choose a time just as the moon rises above the trees in a place that is very quiet.

With your two hands gently cupped, palms face out and raised to the level of your ears as if in a greeting, stand in the Natural Stance with your knees slightly bent. Face the moon for half an hour or longer. You will feel a pressure or a wind blowing into your palms. The best time to do the exercise is when the moon has risen halfway in the sky.

Do not do this exercise in winter unless you are very strong and only in the absence of wind. It is best to perform the Rabbit Salutes the Goddess of Mercy in late spring, summer, and early fall when it is warm. Dress warmly and, if necessary, wear gloves.

This exercise is performed largely for the benefit of your body fluids. It promotes the flow of the Qi in the Yin channels. This Qi is related to all other body fluids.

There is an old Chinese legend about a beautiful lady, Quan Lin, the Lady of Compassion, who lives in the moon. She also represents the feminine principle in the East. Quan Lin has a pet rabbit made of jade. There are many Chinese paintings of this rabbit, who happens to have red eyes, as it stands and faces the moon.

Awakening The Heavenly Eye

Sit cross-legged with your hands in an attitude of prayer. Your eyes should be nearly closed and your attention should be placed on the center of the forehead. Essentially, you are trying to see out of the heavenly eye. If you watch the very tips of your fingers in this pos-

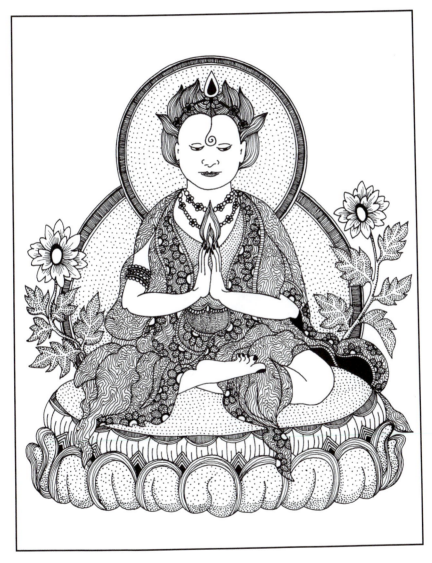

Awakening the Heavenly Eye.

ture (through nearly closed eyes), you may see your Qi as it is emitted from the fingertips. Sitting upright in a chair with your hands in the same attitude will also achieve results.

Leaf Gazing

This exercise does not have its origins in Shaolin Nei Jin Qi Gong. While there may have been other, earlier routes, leaf gazing came to North America by way of a British spiritualist group in the mid 1960s. Gazing is a very good exercise for increasing the ability to see auras. Find a plant you particularly like. Make certain it is not poisonous. Take a leaf from it and place this on a sheet of clean, white paper. In the bright sunlight, sit with the leaf in front of you and gaze.

This is not an exercise in staring. Gazing means to look gently at the leaf, almost through the leaf or "around" it. Study the outer perimeter of the leaf. It is at the junction of the leaf and the paper

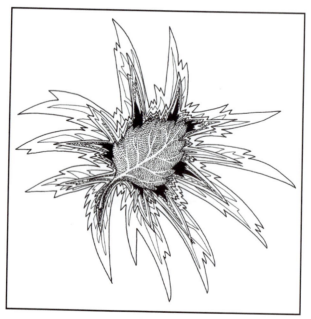

Leaf gazing.

that you will most likely see the aura. After some time, you might notice an unusual glow surrounding the leaf itself. The purpose of the paper is to provide a background so that the aura becomes visible. You will always have better luck leaf gazing in full sunlight.

Concentration

Study the scene in front of your eyes for a few moments. Memorize all possible features. Now close your eyes and hold on to the image in all its detail for five minutes. With practice, try for 10 or 15 minutes. Recall as much detail as you can. This exercise helps both the concentration and the memory, and increases your general level of awareness.

CHAPTER 5

The Channels

Some texts use the term "meridian" to describe the route taken by the Qi as it moves through the body. Following the lead of Kaptchuk, I have used the word "channel." The term "meridian" implies only a two dimensional surface, such as that found on a map, while channel, as in the channel created by a river, includes the third dimension of depth and is therefore a better choice to describe the movement and substance of Qi.

One of the most interesting aspects of any investigation into the nature of the channels is the discovery of the acupuncture points and the meanings of their traditional names. Each name is invested with a detailed meaning, and consequently is an invaluable source of information. The names themselves are rich in metaphor, and often conjure up vivid images about function and relationship. Modern methodology in acupuncture, for practical reasons, typically identifies point names by using numbers associated with channels.

Unfortunately, descriptions such as Governing Vessel (Go. or Du No. 20) do not explain that the ancient name for this point, Baihui, means a "Hundred Reunions." This designation refers to the point's critical role as the confluence of a number of important energetic paths. The energetic effects of stimulating this point through meditation techniques are described in The Crown meditation. A number of the texts in the bibliography describe the related physiological and psychic effects of awakening this and other central points. Any practice will be enriched by a study of these point names. In fact, many of the point names (there are hundreds) are worthy in themselves of a meditation.

For reasons such as these, I have briefly described a few of the points of special interest. Two books have been especially valuable to this study. Arnie Lade's text, *Acupuncture Points: Images & Functions*, discusses the imagery associated with 250 points, while a translation by Michael C. Barnett of an earlier work by Jean-Claude Darras, *Traité d'Acuponcture Médicale, Tombe 1* discusses, in some detail, the meaning and energetics associated with most of the points on the Regular and Strange Channels.

An ancient saying states that, "If you open your mouth or move your hands in an attempt to heal without a knowledge of channels, then you will inevitably make mistakes." Another says, "Being a medical doctor without a knowledge of the channels is like working in the dark without a light." Knowledge of these channels and their associated acupuncture points is of paramount importance for Qi Gong practitioners. Understanding these pathways enables us to envision the Qi as it moves in its circuitous route and to see complex relationships between the organs and tissues in the body.

In Chinese acupuncture, channels are called "Jing Luo." Jing refers to the main vertical channels and Luo refers to the side branches which run horizontally. Together they comprise the network of channels running everywhere through the body. There are 12 main vertical or Regular Channels, 15 main horizontal or Collateral Channels, and eight Strange or Extra Channels. Two of the Strange Channels, the Ren and the Du Channels, are grouped with the 12 Regular Channels, making 14 in all. Each of these 14 channels has its own Collateral Channel, as does the spleen, making up the 15 altogether. The 12 Regular Channels are either Yin or Yang in character, and are associated with either the foot or the hand, depending on their point of origin or ending.

The Yin channels are termed the Taiyin, Shaoyin, and Jueyin. There are three Yin hand channels and these are connected to the lungs, the heart, and the pericardium (which, in Traditional Chinese Medicine, is considered an independent organ.) There are also three Yin foot channels, and these are connected to the spleen, the kidneys, and the liver. The Yin channels are connected to Yin organs which are understood to be solid. These six organs are collectively referred to as Zang organs and their primary purpose is to produce and store vital essence, Qi, blood and other body fluids.

The three Yang channels are the Yangming, Taiyang, and Shaoyang. Three Yang hand channels are connected to the large intestine, small intestine, and the Triple Burner. Another three Yang foot channels are connected to the stomach, bladder, and gallbladder. These Yang channels are connected to the hollow, Yang, organs (mentioned just above) and are referred to as Fu organs. The central purpose of Fu organs is to process food, assimilate nutrients, and eliminate wastes. Two other extraordinary organs, the brain and the uterus, are also Fu organs.

Table 6: Key to Symbols.

- - - - - - - - - - - - -	Channel inside the body
————————	Channel on the surface of the body
●	Acupuncture point
Δ	Acupuncture point (crossing point) belonging to a different channel
X X # 1	A numbering system corresponding to specific acupuncture points on a specified channel

All channels have bilateral symmetry (not shown) except for the Governing Vessel (Du, page 160) and the Conception (Ren, page 162) channels.

Together, these organs are linked through the vast systems of channels to form the Zang-Fu network. It is this complex which enables practitioners of Traditional Chinese Medicine to regard and treat the human body as an integrated whole, and to identify relationships where none appear to exist. Each of the hand and foot pairs mentioned above are closely related, so that bending fingers also affects the foot channels. The stomach, for example, is affected at the same time as the large intestine. This association simplifies our practice.

For the purposes of our practice, only the 12 Regular Channels and four of the Strange Channels will be discussed. When examining the channel diagrams, remember that bilateral symmetry of the channels is assumed even though the diagrams represent the points on only one side of the body. Table 6 on page 129 provides a key to the symbols used on the figures.

The Twelve Regular Channels

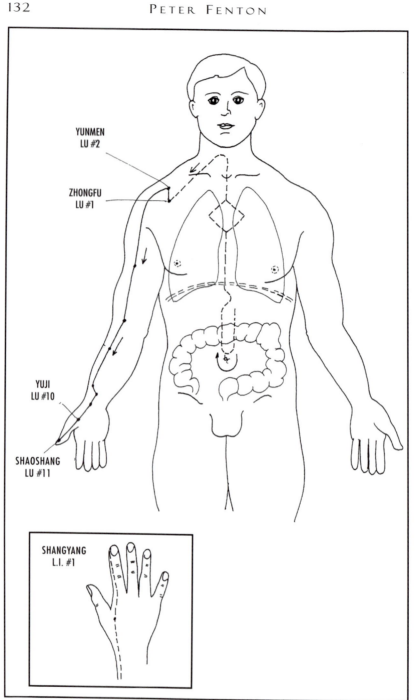

The Lung Channel of the Hand Taiyin.

THE LUNG CHANNEL OF THE HAND TAIYIN

The channel (page 133) begins in the middle of the stomach, moves downward to connect the large intestine, then up to its pertinent organ, the lungs. From here, it moves through the throat, appearing at the Zhongfu point Lu. No. 1. Then it moves up to the Yunmen point Lu. No. 2, and then downward across the shoulder, down the arm, through the wrist to the Yuji point Lu. No. 10 on the thumb, ending at the Shaoshang point Lu. No. 11. Here it links with the Large Intestine Channel of the Hand Yangming. If you are working on lung problems, treatment can begin here.

Translated, Zhongfu means "Central Dwelling" as in an administrative center. The channel, itself, appears from within the body cavity at this point, having traveled through the Triple Burner regions. It is closely linked to the circulation of Qi through all the channels. The Yunmen point means the "Gate of the Clouds." This point is the exit for the vapors created by the heating function of the Triple Burner (hence its name.) The Yuji point means "Border of the Fish," a reference to a prominent anatomical feature in the thumb. Shaoshang means the "Young Exchange." It indicates the source point of an energy exchange between this point, the ending of the Lung Channel, and the next point, the Shangyang, meaning "Exchange of Yang," which begins the Large Intestine (L.I.) Channel.

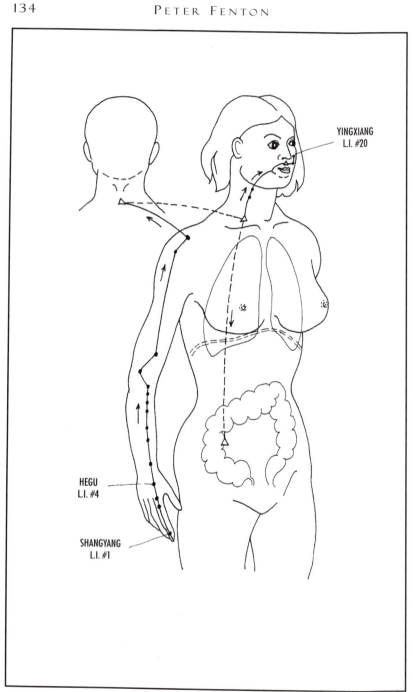

The Large Intestine Channel of the Hand Yangming.

THE LARGE INTESTINE CHANNEL
OF THE HAND YANGMING

The channel (page 134) begins at the point Shangyang, L.I. No. 1 , on the index finger, travels up the side of the index finger, through the Hegu point L.I. No. 4, along the forearm to the elbow, further up the upper arm and detours over the back of the top of the arm to the base of the neck. Then it moves through the body to the clavicular region, where it communicates with the lung. Here it branches, one section moving downward through the diaphragm to the large intestines.

The other moves upward through the neck and cheek and into the gums of the lower molars and teeth. It moves across to the upper lip and meets with its counterpart on the other side of the body at the Renzhong point on the Du Channel No. 26, at the midpoint of the groove in the upper lip. (This point is used for descriptive purposes and is not associated with this particular channel.) The paths cross over and move upward along the sides of nostrils, to the Yingxiang point L.I. No. 20, beside the nose.

The Yingxiang point, meaning "Reception of Odors," is used to treat sneezing, facial paralysis or the nose in general. Note that pinching the Renzhong point, meaning "Philtrum," can restore someone who has fainted. The Shangyang point, explained above, is used to treat toothache, sore throat, numbness of fingers, and loss of consciousness. Hegu means the "Convergence of Valleys" and is located just below the intersection of the thumb and first finger. The name is a reference to its anatomical location. It is used to treat the throat, large intestine, shortness of breath, colds, or flu.

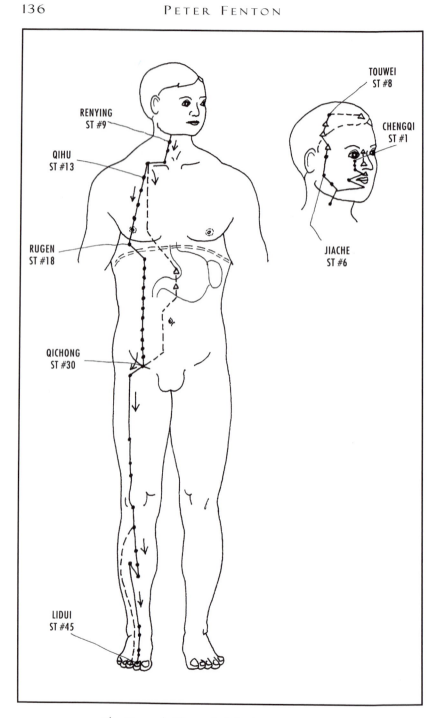

RENYING
ST #9

QIHU
ST #13

RUGEN
ST #18

QICHONG
ST #30

LIDUI
ST #45

TOUWEI
ST #8

CHENGQI
ST #1

JIACHE
ST #6

The Stomach Channel of the Foot Yangming.

STOMACH CHANNEL
OF THE FOOT YANGMING

The channel (page 136) begins at the Yingxiang point (which is the L.I. point No. 20) on both sides of the nose and rises to the bridge. It moves downward along the side of the nose through the Chengqi point Stomach (St. No. 1), enters the upper gums, moves around the lips to the Jiache point, St. No. 6. The channel moves around the jaw, and branches part of the way along the line of the jaw. One branch continues past the ear to the Touwei point, St. No. 8, just above the hairline. This point is used to treat migraines, one-sided headaches, and the blurring of vision.

This branch continues downward to the navel, where it enters the Qichong point, St. No. 30, on the lower abdomen in the interior of the body. Here, the two original channels meet.

The second branch moves down to the Renying point, St. No. 9. It continues its descent passing through the throat. At the Qihu point, St. No. 13, on the clavicle, an interior passage branches off to pass through the diaphragm and enters the stomach. A lateral branch separates here to connect with the spleen. The main branch continues its descent to the Rugen point, St. No. 18, and down the Qichong point where the two branches meet. Moving downward, the channel passes along the thigh, past the knee, through the ankle, and ends at the Lidui point, St. No. 45, on the second toe near the nail.

Chenqi refers to the "Place which Receives Tears." It has been used for a variety of eye problems, including myopia, night blindness, and spasms of the eye. The Jiache point is an anatomical reference to the maxilla (jaw bone). Towei is another reference to an anatomical feature, this time to the coronal suture on the cranium. This point has been used for headache, blurring of vision, and vertigo.

The Renying point, interpreted as "Meeting with Man," is applied for hypertension, sore throats, and asthma. Qihu means "Door of Energy." It is here that Qi enters the interior of the chest. It can be used to treat bronchitis, asthma, and hiccup. Rugen is another reference to anatomy, this time to the "Base of the Breast." The Qichong point, meaning "Assault of Energy," is used to treat genital diseases, irregular menstruation and hernia. The Lidui point, meaning "Controlled Exchange," is used to treat toothaches, dream-disturbed sleep, mental confusion, and fevers. Since it is the terminal point in the channel, it is also the point of exchange with the next channel.

SPLEEN CHANNEL
OF THE FOOT TAIYIN

The channel (page 139) begins at the tip of the big toe, and travels up the inside of the foot and leg to the abdomen. Here it connects with the spleen and the stomach. It continues through the diaphragm and then moves to the throat. At the root of the tongue, it spreads out.

This channel is very important in acupuncture. The Yinbai point, Spleen (Sp. No. 1), which begins this channel, means "Hidden Clarity" (referring to its effects on the thinking process), or "Hidden White" (referring to the whiteness of the flesh where it is located). Found on the big toe near the cuticle of the nail, it is used for abdominal distention, uterine bleeding, and dream-disturbed sleep. The Lougu point Sp. No. 7, or "Sleeping Valley," is used for cold, numbness, and paralysis of the leg and knee. The Xuehai point Sp. No. 10, known as the "Sea of Blood," is located above the knee on the inside of the leg. As its name implies, it is used to treat any blood-related problems, such as hypertension, or irregular and abnormal menstrual cycles. Essentially, it is used in the regulation and distribution of the blood. The Dabao point Sp. No. 21 translates as the "Great Envelope." From this point, blood and Nutritional Qi, which later "envelop the body," are distributed. It is used to treat asthma and general weakness.

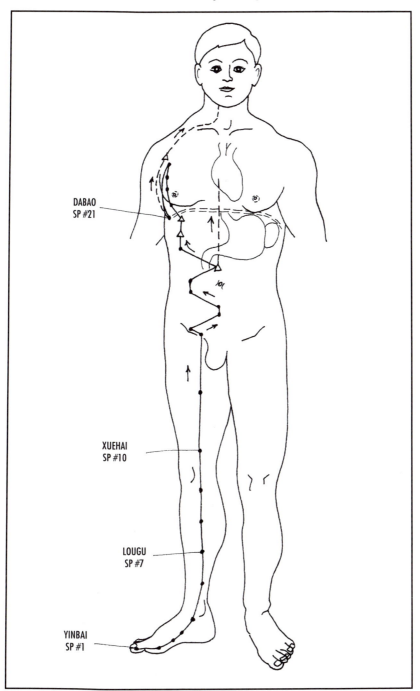

DABAO
SP #21

XUEHAI
SP #10

LOUGU
SP #7

YINBAI
SP #1

The Spleen Channel of the Foot Taiyin.

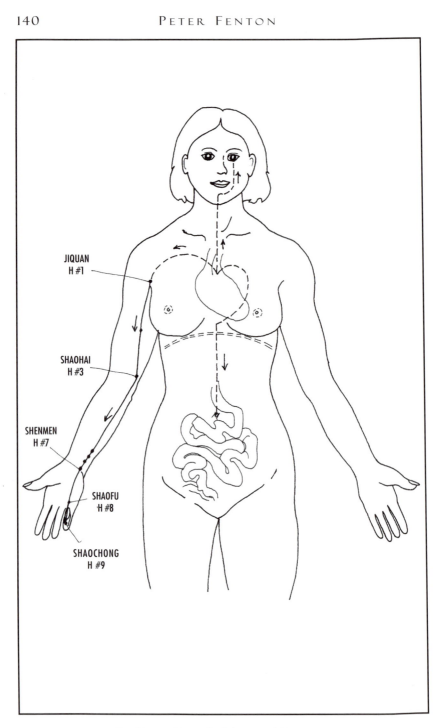

JIQUAN
H #1

SHAOHAI
H #3

SHENMEN
H #7

SHAOFU
H #8

SHAOCHONG
H #9

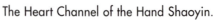

The Heart Channel of the Hand Shaoyin.

HEART CHANNEL
OF THE HAND SHAOYIN

The channel (page 140) finds its origins in the heart. It passes through the heart system to connect with the vessels joining the heart to the other Zang-Fu organs. Then it moves down through the diaphragm into the small intestine. Another branch ascends along the throat to the tissues surrounding the eyes. A final channel moves from the heart to the lungs to the Jiquan point Heart (H. No. 1), the inside of the arm, and then down the arm to the Shaohai point H. No. 3, on the inner side of the elbow. It continues through the Shenmen point H. No. 7 on the wrist, the Shaofu point H. No. 8 on the palm, and ends at the Shaochong point H. No. 9 on the little finger, near the root of the nail.

Depending on who you consult, Jiquan can mean either "Extreme Source," or "Summit's Spring." Here the Qi wells to the surface of the body, like the bubbling of an underground spring. It regulates the heart and has been used for arthritis in the shoulder, and pains in the heart, elbow, and arm. The Shaohai point suggests a Young or Lesser Sea. Traditionally, this point was used to calm the heart. It is also used for numbness of the forearm, elbow diseases, as well as cardiac pains. Shenmen identifies a Qi gate or doorway, through which the Spirit can be affected. Its central function is as a tonic for heart and Spirit, and to regulate the channels.

The Shaofu point is used for aphasia[1] (due to hysteria), pain in the chest, enuresis, and toothache. Its name suggests a secondary residence where the Qi gathers before it moves on, in this case to the Shaochong point, meaning "Lesser Rushing," "Lesser Pouring," or "Young Assault" (depending on who is consulted), which is the ending point of the channel. It is here that the Qi from the channel rushes into (assaults) the next channel. It has been used for severe fever, coma, cardiac pain, depression, hysteria, and has also been used in cases involving loss of consciousness, and even insanity.

---

1. Aphasia = loss of speech.

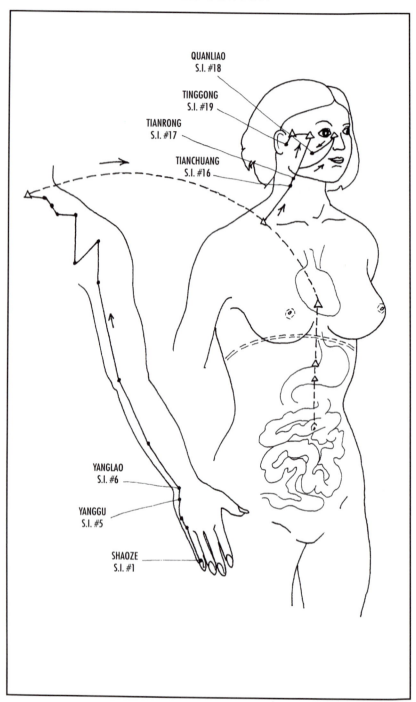

QUANLIAO
S.I. #18

TINGGONG
S.I. #19

TIANRONG
S.I. #17

TIANCHUANG
S.I. #16

YANGLAO
S.I. #6

YANGGU
S.I. #5

SHAOZE
S.I. #1

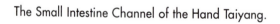

The Small Intestine Channel of the Hand Taiyang.

THE SMALL INTESTINE CHANNEL OF THE HAND TAIYANG

The channel (page 142) begins at the Shaoze point, Small Intestine (S.I. No. 1) at the outside tip of the little finger. Moving upward through the wrist, it passes through the Yanggu S.I. No. 5 and Yanglao points S.I. No. 6. It then moves along the outside of the arm, up to the back of the shoulder, and traverses the shoulder blade to the collarbone. Here, one channel connects to the heart. It then descends along the esophagus and through the diaphragm to the stomach, and lastly to the small intestine, its pertinent organ. The other channel moves from the collar bone area up the side of the neck through the Tianchuang S.I. No. 16 and Tianrong S.I. No. 17 points, to the Quanliao S.I. No. 18 point on the cheek. It then branches to the ear and ends at the Tinggong point S.I. No. 19, in front of the ear.

The Shaoze point translates as "Young" or "Lesser Marsh." Here the Qi accumulates, cools, and is moistened, as if it were in a marsh, before it continues on its course. It is used for mastitis, lactation deficiency, headache, and sore throat. For shoulder pains, emit Qi on this point (at the root of the nail), and then again on the channel points on the back of the shoulder.

The Yanglao point, which means "Nourishing the Aged," is known for its ability to refresh the Yang Qi. The effect is, essentially, rejuvenation. It is used for joint pains in the shoulder, neck, and back, and for blurring of vision. Tianchuang means "Heaven's Window." Here the Qi is about to enter into the Heavenly region of the body, the head. Tianrong, the following point, suggests a "Glimpse of Heaven" or the "Contents of Heaven." The Qi from the lower reaches of the body now becomes involved with higher processes. The point is stimulated for deafness, swellings in the neck, tinnitus, and asthma.

As the name suggests, the Tinggong point, or "Listening Palace," has been used for tinnitus, deafness, and inflammation of the ear. It has also been used for toothache and facial paralysis. For tinnitus, press the point gently with your middle finger and exhale slowly for one minute after practicing Qi Gong. For more serious cases, center your palms over the point several inches away. Move your hands in a spiral manner outward and away from the ears. Then, when your palms are two feet away, reverse direction.

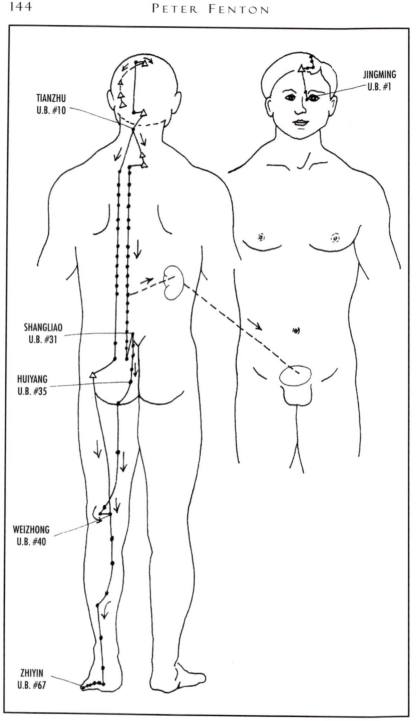

The Urinary Bladder Channel of the Foot Taiyang.

URINARY BLADDER CHANNEL
OF THE FOOT TAIYANG

This is a large channel accommodating 67 points. The channel (page 144) begins inside the eye socket at the Jingming point Urinary Bladder (U.B. No. 1). It rises to the forehead, where a branch moves to the temple. Another part penetrates and communicates with the brain. It leaves the brain from the posterior and forks at the Tianzhu point U.B. No. 10: both channels run downward, flanking the spinal column. The Shangliao point U.B. No. 31 and the Huiyang point U.B. No. 35 are points of interest in the region of the lower spine.

One channel enters the body and connects with the kidney and the urinary bladder. Both continue their descent to the thigh, and meet at the Weizhong point U.B. No. 40 at the back of the knee joint. The channel ends at the Zhiyin point U.B. No. 67, on the outside tip of the little toe. This channel is used to treat urinary and kidney problems, eye pain, headaches, backaches, chills, fever, and leg problems. This is one of the most important channels, since it covers the entire length of the body. The Jingming point means "Clarity of the Eye," and is used for night and color blindness, and other eye problems. Tianzhu means "Pillar of Heaven," a point name reflecting its strategic position on the back of the neck, reflecting its strategic position of supporting the head.

The Shangliao, an anatomical reference to the first sacral vertebra, can be used for such diverse ailments as lower back pain, constipation, prolapsed uterus, and irregular menstruation. The name Huiyang means "Meeting of the Yang" and indicates its energetic character. Here the Yang Qi gathers at the base of the spine. It is used to treat difficulties with the sexual organs, dysentery, and hemorrhoids. Use the other points along the side of the sacrum to treat sciatica, lower back, and leg pain.

The two points on the knee, the Weiyang, and the Weizhong (both points refer to their anatomical location) are used to treat leg problems. The final point on the channel, Zhiyin, means "Point of Extreme Yin." It is used for various problems, such as difficult labor, head and neck aches, and blockages of the nasal passage. Qi passes through this point before moving into the kidney channel.

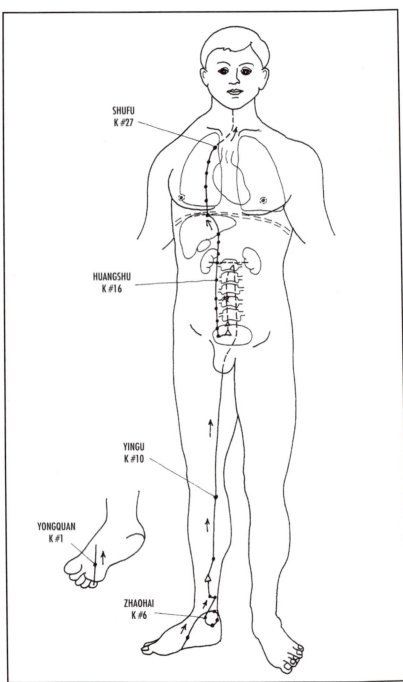

The Kidney Channel of the Foot Shaoyin.

THE KIDNEY CHANNEL
OF THE FOOT SHAOYIN

This is another important channel. When using cold Qi to treat patients, they often feel a cold sensation blowing out the bottom of the foot, as if a wind was moving through them. The channel (page 146) begins at the little toe, moves to the Yongquan point Kidney (K. No. 1) at the top of the sole in the center of the foot. It moves around the ankle and into the heel, passing through the Zhaohai point K. No. 6. Then it follows the inside of the leg, moving through the Yingu point K. No. 10 to the top of the thigh, where it enters the base of the spinal column. It rises through the Huangshu point K. No. 16 to the kidney, and joins with the urinary bladder.

One branch passes through the liver and the diaphragm to enter the lungs and throat. The other branch leaves the lungs to join with the heart and chest. The main channel continues its rise through the Shufu point K. No. 27, on the lower edge of the collarbone. Although this is the last actual point on the channel, it continues its rise to end at the root of the tongue.

Yongquan means "Gushing Spring," and is suggestive of living waters flowing upward into the body. Massaging this point will promote the flow of Qi entering, or leaving, the body. This channel can be used to treat hypertension, but should not be used by those with low blood pressure. The Zhaohai point translates as "Luminous or Shining Sea," and reflects the function of this point, which is to serve as a reservoir for Qi when it is in a particularly vigorous state. It is used for many purposes, such as hernia, insomnia, and sore throat, but derives much of its significance from its ability to cool excessive fire in the body and to calm the Spirit.

The Yingu point is a reference to the energetics of the point, and means "Valley of Yin." It is used for urinary problems, impotence, and arthritic pains in the knee. Located adjacent to the navel, Huangshu means "Vitals' Hollow," and refers to the vital center of the cardio-diaphragmatic region.

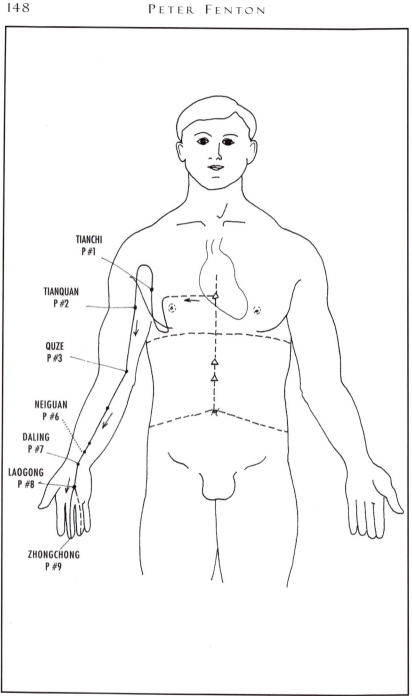

TIANCHI
P #1

TIANQUAN
P #2

QUZE
P #3

NEIGUAN
P #6

DALING
P #7

LAOGONG
P #8

ZHONGCHONG
P #9

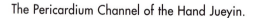

The Pericardium Channel of the Hand Jueyin.

THE PERICARDIUM CHANNEL OF THE HAND JUEYIN

This channel (page 148) begins in the chest. One branch connects to the pericardium and then descends through the three layers of the Triple Burner, known as the upper, middle, and lower Jiao, or collectively as the Sanjiao.

Another branch extends out through the Tianchi point Pericardium (P. No. 1) near the nipple. Then it moves to the upper arm and downward through the Tianquan point P. No. 2, along the inside of the arm, through the Quze point P. No. 3, just above the elbow. The channel continues its descent through the Daling point P. No. 7 on the wrist to the Laogong point P. No. 8 on the palm, and further to the Zhongchong point P. No. 9 at the tip of the middle finger.

The heart region, because of its vital functions and role as a command center, is assigned an association with "Heaven" similar to that of the head. For this reason point No. 1 is called Tianchi, "Heaven's or Celestial Pool." Tianquan is closely allied with the first point, and means "Heaven's or Celestial Source" of pure Qi. The Daling point, or "Big Mound," near the crease of the wrist and the Neiguan point, or "Inner Gate," have both been used to relieve irregular heartbeat, nausea, motion sickness, mental disorders, and epilepsy. The term "Inner Gate" refers to this point's role as a gateway to other channels in the region.

The Laogong point, or "Palace of Labor," evokes the association of the hand with physical work. It is important when treating others and is frequently used. If you are emitting Qi through this point, you are also emitting through the equivalent point on the sole of your foot so that, in theory, you can treat with your feet, as well. The terminal point of the channel, Zhongchong, means "Middle Rushing" or "Middle Pouring." Here the Qi from the channel pours into the body from the surface. Middle not only refers to the point's location on the middle finger, but also to its location between the more superficial Taiyin and the deeper Shaoyin Channels of the arm.

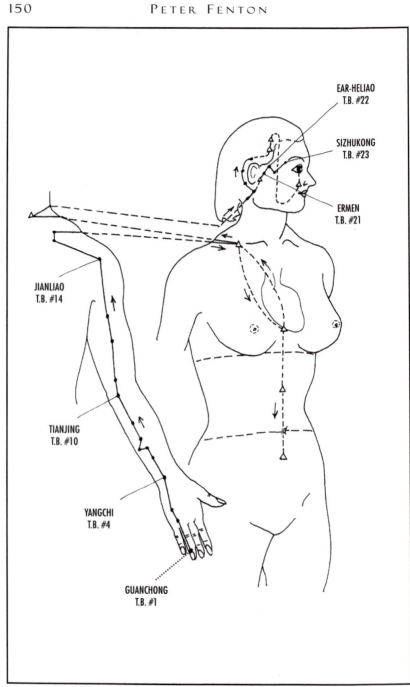

EAR-HELIAO
T.B. #22

SIZHUKONG
T.B. #23

ERMEN
T.B. #21

JIANLIAO
T.B. #14

TIANJING
T.B. #10

YANGCHI
T.B. #4

GUANCHONG
T.B. #1

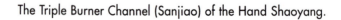

The Triple Burner Channel (Sanjiao) of the Hand Shaoyang.

THE TRIPLE BURNER CHANNEL (SANJIAO) OF THE HAND SHAOYANG

This channel (page 150) begins at the Guanchong point Triple Burner (T.B. No. 1) on the ring finger, just above the nail on the outside of the finger. It moves through the hand to the Yangchi point T.B. No. 4 on the wrist at the back of the hand. Continuing upward, it passes through the Tianjing point T.B. No. 10 on the back of the elbow to the Jianliao point T.B. No. 14 on the back of the shoulder. It then moves through the chest and pericardium to the upper, middle, and lower parts of the Triple Burner.

A branch, originating in the chest, moves to the shoulder and neck to the Ermen T.B. No. 21 and Ear-Heliao T.B. No. 22, points next to the inside of the ear, and then to the Sizhukong point T.B. No. 23 at the outer edge of the eyebrow. Beneath the ear, another branch moves around the outside of the ear up to a point on the side of the forehead. Here it descends, moving around the cheek, then up past the side of the nose to the lower eyelid.

The Guanchong point is interpreted as the "Gate's Pouring." As a result of its vigor, at this point the Qi is capable of penetrating the barrier or gate, and so it moves into this channel from the internal regions. It is used in treating headaches, irritability, sore throat, and problems with speech. The anatomical location of the Yangchi point in a hollow on the wrist serves as a location for the Yang Qi to pool. Its name, "Pool of Yang," reflects its purpose. It is used for regional pains in wrist, shoulder, arm, malaria, and deafness.

The Tianjing point in the elbow, meaning "Celestial Well," alludes to this point's capacity as a reservoir, supplying the "Heavens" with Qi. It is used for problems with lower chest, neck, shoulder, and arm. The Jianliao point is found in a depression, and its name, "Shoulder Opening" or "Shoulder Seam," reflects this location. It is used in shoulder-related conditions.

At the Ermen point, or "Gate of the Ear," the Qi leaves the ear. It is used for ear and hearing-related difficulties such as deafness, tinnitus, and ear infections. It can also be useful with toothaches.

The Ear-Heliao is a reference to an anatomical feature, and it is used in much the same way as the Ermen point, but can also be used for lockjaw. Sizhukong refers to the "Silken Bamboo Hollow," which is the bamboo-shaped hollow which accommodates the eye. Stimulating this point affects twitching eyelids, facial paralysis, color and night blindness, and conjunctivitis.

GALLBLADDER CHANNEL OF THE FOOT SHAOYANG

Interestingly, this channel has 20 points in the head alone. After some practice all 10 fingers emit Qi, so you can treat this channel by running your fingers through the hair. The channel (page 154) begins at the outer edge of the eye at the Tongziliao point Gallbladder (G.B.)No. 1), and travels in a complicated route around the head passing through the Qubin point G.B. No. 7 above the ear, the Benshen point G.B. No. 13 on the forehead, the Yangbai point G.B. No. 14, also on the forehead above the eyebrow, and the Fengchi point G.B. No. 20 on the neck.

Two branches travels down through the chest, liver, gallbladder, along the outside of the leg, and meet at the Huantiao point G.B. No. 30. The channel continues to descend through the Yanglingquan point G.B. No. 34, to the Qiuxu point in the ankle at G.B. 40, and on to the end of the toe at the Foot (or Zu) Qiaoyin G.B. No. 44.

Tongziliao means the "Pupil's Seam," and refers to the bony surface beside the eye. It is used for headaches, ametropia (any abnormal condition of the refraction of the eye), and night blindness. Qubin is another anatomical reference to a point at the "Crook of the Temple." This is used for migraine headache and lockjaw. The Benshen point, meaning "Original Spirit," has an important connection with activities of the brain and mind, hence its usefulness in treating seizures, hemiplegia (paralysis of one side of the body), headache, and blurring of vision.

The name Yangbai, or "Yang White," pertains to its function of healing the eyes and restoring them by infusing them with Yang Qi. It is used to treat sore eyes, conjunctivitis, twitching eyelids, frontal headaches, and night blindness. The last point on the head, Fengchi, is explained as "Pool of Wind." Traditionally, this is the point where the Wind can attack and deposit "Evil Qi" in the body. It pools here before moving deeper into the body.

The Huantiao point on the buttocks means "Encircling Leap." Traditionally, a successful treatment of this channel evoked a mus-

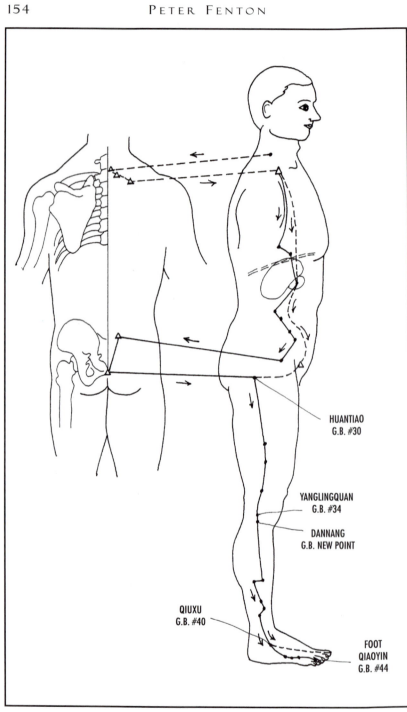

HUANTIAO
G.B. #30

YANGLINGQUAN
G.B. #34

DANNANG
G.B. NEW POINT

QIUXU
G.B. #40

FOOT
QIAOYIN
G.B. #44

The Gallbladder Channel of the Foot Shaoyang.

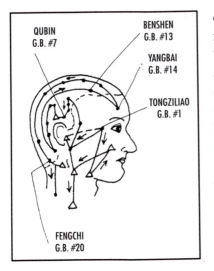

QUBIN
G.B. #7

BENSHEN
G.B. #13

YANGBAI
G.B. #14

TONGZILIAO
G.B. #1

FENGCHI
G.B. #20

cular reaction, therefore its name. Yang-lingquan means "Yang Mound Spring" and is an anatomical reference to the head of the fibula, a bone on the inside of the leg. It is useful in treating hip, knee, and leg disorders, and has been used for many other purposes, including constipation, incontinence, hepatitis, and driving unhealthy Qi (including anger) from the liver. It is especially useful when working with the gallbladder.

Qiuxu means "Mound of Ruins" and refers to the "mound" at the ankle. It is applied to relieve pain and some diseases in the chest, ribs, lower back, ankles, colic, and inflammation of the lymphatic glands. The foot Qiaoyin translates as "Yin Cavity of the Foot." Here the Qi from the channel moves out of the Gallbladder Channel and into the (Yin) Liver Channel. It is useful in treating asthma, pleurisy, hypertension, difficulties in breathing, and headache.

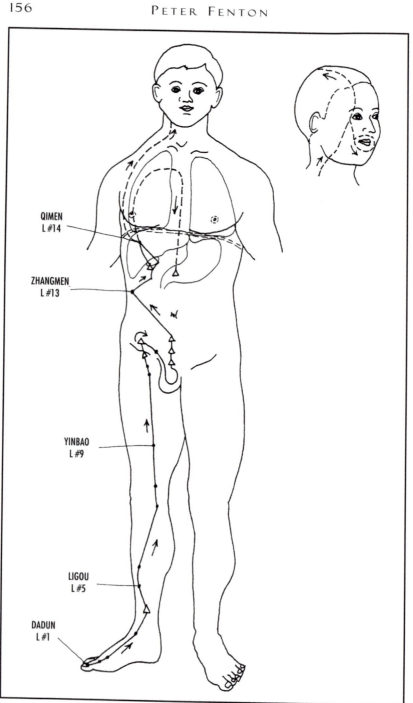

The Liver Channel of the Foot Jueyin.

LIVER CHANNEL
OF THE FOOT JUEYIN

The channel (page 156) has 14 points. It begins on the inside of the
big toe behind the nail at the Dadun point, Liver (L. No. 1). Moving
along the upper surface of the foot, it rises up the inside of the leg
through the Ligou point L. No. 5 and the Yinbao point L. No. 9, to
the pubic region. Here it circles the genitals. It moves upward to
the lower abdomen and stomach. Next, it enters the liver and communicates with the gallbladder. Continuing its rise, one branch
moves to the diaphragm and lower chest. The main branch further
ascends along the trachea to connect with the tissues around the
eyes, cheeks, lips, and the forehead. It terminates at the Du
Channel. The lower branch begins in the liver and moves through
the diaphragm, ending in the lungs.

This channel is used to treat conditions of the liver and gall
bladder, and has some influence over the lungs, stomach, and
brain. The coloration of the eyes is one indication of the condition
of the liver. The liver is also a well-known repository for negative
emotions. "Anger hurts the liver," and "Depression hurts the
spleen," are two well-known expressions. A peaceful mind, con-
versely, is conducive to the health of the organs and inner
processes.

The Dadun point means point of "Great Calmness" and has
been used to treat prolapsed uterus, hernia, and enuresis. The
Ligou point translates as the "Drain of Shells," a reference to an
ancient Taoist tradition of using a specific shell to measure water
taken from the sea. Water taken in this way was regarded as pure.
The reference here, then, is to the pure quality of energy found at
this point. It is used to treat menstrual difficulties, dysuria (difficult
or painful urination), and leg pains.

Zhangmen, L. point No. 13, means "System's Door" or "Gate
of the Section." This title refers to the capacity of the point to favorably influence the Yin organs since it is situated at their confluence.
It can be used to treat jaundice, certain types of diarrhea, vomiting,
and constipation.

The last point on the channel, Qimen L. No. 14, translates to mean "Expectation's Door" or "The Gate of Hope." The name refers to the cyclical nature of the energy moving through this gate. The reference is to the periodic nature of the flow of Qi through this gate. It has particular relevance during the menstrual cycle when stagnating energy is retained in the reproductive center. Since stagnating liver Qi can result in depression, working with this point can have psychologically beneficial results. This point has also been used to treat hepatitis, cirrhosis of the liver, enlarged liver, chest pains, pleurisy, and hiccup.

The Strange Channels

There are eight channels that are referred to as Strange or Extraordinary because they travel in unusual patterns through the body. These eight do not relate to any specific organs as do the other 12. And, with the exception of the Governing and Conception Channels, they do not have any acupuncture points of their own, but use those of other channels. Four Strange Channels are discussed briefly here because of their importance to our practice.

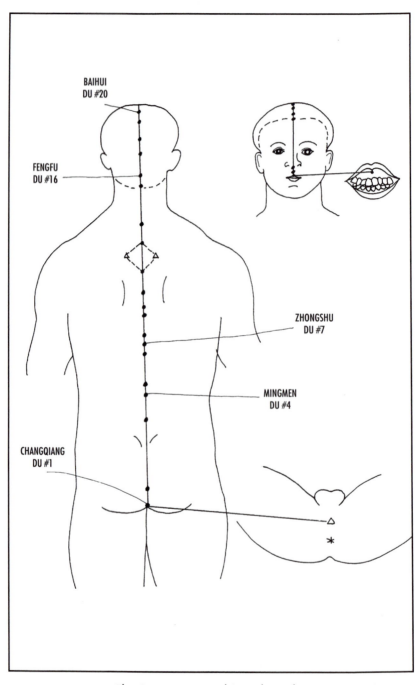

BAIHUI
DU #20

FENGFU
DU #16

ZHONGSHU
DU #7

MINGMEN
DU #4

CHANGQIANG
DU #1

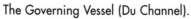

The Governing Vessel (Du Channel).

THE GOVERNING CHANNEL
(DU CHANNEL)

The Governing Vessel or Du Channel (page 160) is Yang in nature. There are 28 points along its course. It begins at the Changqiang point Du No. 1 between the anus and the coccyx. It rises straight up the back along the inside of the spinal vertebrae through the Mingmen Du No. 4 and the Zhongshu Du No. 7. Continuing, it passes through the Fengfu point Du No. 16, where it enters the brain. The main channel rises over the cranium along the center of the forehead, to the bridge of the nose, and the gums above the front teeth. The Baihui point Du No. 20 at the crown has been discussed earlier.

The Changqiang point means "Long" or "Lasting Strength." It plays a vital role, and its name refers to the energy associated with this point. It has been used to treat prolapsed anus, hemorrhoids, and lower back pain. Mingmen means "Life Gate" or "Gate of Vitality," and has been used for spinal problems, asthma, epilepsy, and febrile diseases. In our practice it provides a conduit whereby we can replenish our energies. A passage in the Life Gate Meditation discusses the gate at some length.

Zhongshu or "Central Hinge" has special importance as the focal point for the Triple Burner. It has been used as a tonic for the spine and for digestive problems. Fengfu means the "Dwelling of the Wind." Wind, in this sense, refers to external pathogenic energy. It accumulates at this point before continuing its path into your body. Its uses are varied and it has been used to treat mental disease, hemiplegia, stiff neck, and the aftereffects of apoplexy.

The Baihui point, as discussed at the beginning of the chapter, is a very important Qi gate. When it opens, you will have achieved a breakthrough in your practice. If you are seated in a darkened room, it is possible to see a pillar of gold, white, or purple light radiating forth to the ceiling. It is commonly used by acupuncturists to produce anesthesia, thereby preparing a patient for brain surgery.

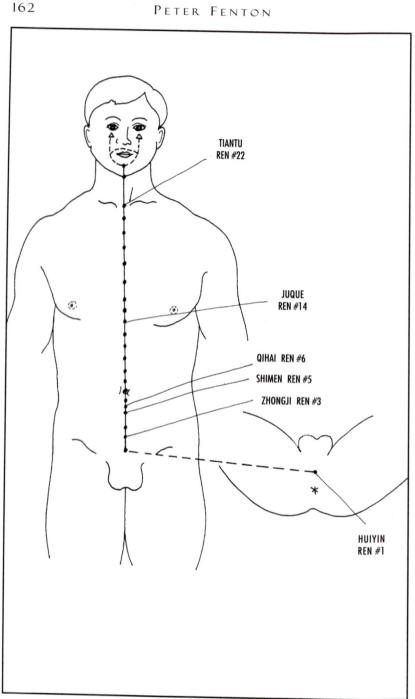

The Conception Vessel (Ren Channel).

THE CONCEPTION CHANNEL (REN CHANNEL)

This channel (page 162) starts at the Huiyin point Ren No. 1 at the perineum, and rises along the centerline of the body through the Zhongji point, Ren No. 3, in the abdomen. It continues through the stomach, chest, and throat, passing through the Shimen point Ren No. 5, the Qihai point Ren No. 6, the Juque point Ren No. 14, and the Tiantu point, Ren No. 22. Branching to both sides of the face, it moves around the lips, through the cheeks, and terminates just below the center of the eyes.

Huiyin point means "Reunion" or "Meeting of the Yin." It refers to the fact that three of the Strange Channels, the Conception, the Governing, and the Vital Channels, meet here. A number of the exercises, especially those involving the Horse Stance, rely on this point to enable the flow of Qi in the body. Zhongzi is a term which translates as "Middle Summit" or "Central Extremity." Here the three Yin channels of the lower limbs, the Liver, Spleen, and Kidney, reunite.

Shimen means "Gate of Stone." An infertile woman in China is sometimes spoken of as a "Woman of Stone." The term may have developed as a result of the ancient Chinese writings which indicated that puncturing this point might actually cause sterility. As a result, the classical texts prohibit the use of needles with this point. This point is also held to be very important by some schools for strengthening personal Qi and for accumulating inner strength. Many exercises affect this point including "Holding the Ball with Two Hands."

Qihai means "Sea of Qi." The Qi gathers here, after entering the body through the Shimen point, like water flowing from the rivers to the ocean. This point is especially important to the regulation and rejuvenation of the Qi. It has been used for many physical ailments including insomnia, intestinal paralysis, urinary dysfunctions, chronic diarrhea, and irregular menstruation.

Tiantu has been translated as both "Heaven's Chimney" and "Celestial Prominence." Its location, at the juncture of the chest and neck, gives it its association with the heavens and the "Chimney" or "Prominence" is an anatomical reference to the trachea. The point is particularly useful for diseases of the chest and throat, such as coughs, asthma, sore throat, bronchitis, common colds, and chest pains.

THE BELT CHANNEL
(DAI CHANNEL)

This channel (page 165) is the only Strange Channel that moves horizontally. It travels in a path roughly indicated by its name. Because of the Belt's proximity and relation to side channels, most Qi Gong exercises begin with the Horse or Natural Stance to awaken it. This indicates its great importance. The Belt has three points along its course, all of which belong to the Gallbladder Channel: the Daimai point G.B. No. 26, the Wushu point G.B. No. 27, and the Weidaoc point G.B. No. 28. Each of these names has some special reference to the point's ability to work within the Belt Channel.

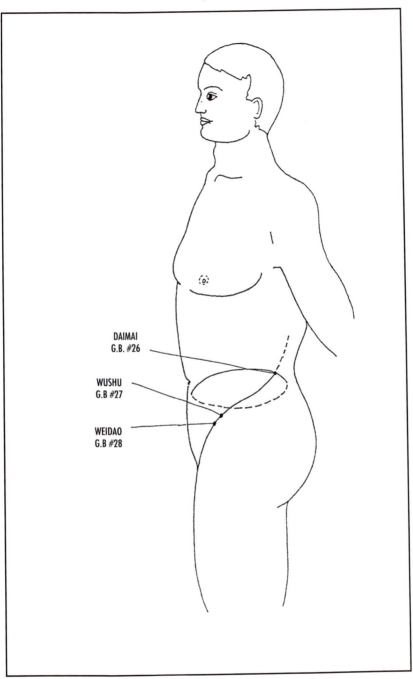

DAIMAI
G.B. #26

WUSHU
G.B #27

WEIDAO
G.B #28

The Belt Channel (Dai Channel).

THE VITAL CHANNEL
(CHONG CHANNEL)

This channel (page 167) begins in the lower abdomen, descends and appears at the perineum. After this point, it rises inside the vertebrae. A second branch passes through the Qichong point on the Stomach Channel and then intersects with the Kidney Channel, rising through the throat and upper lips.

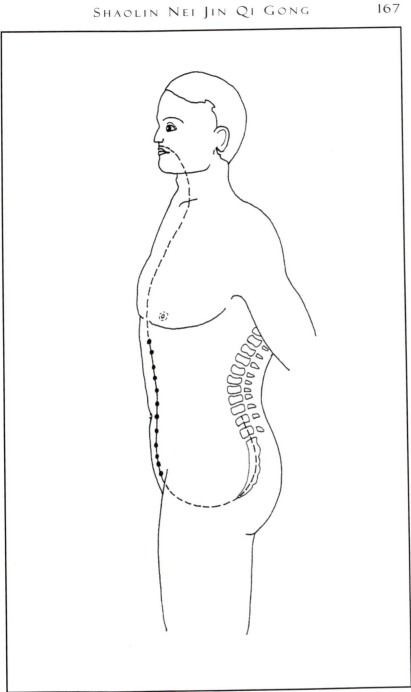

The Vital Channel (Chong Channel).

Annotated Bibliography

Arnold, Sir Edwin, trans. *The Song Celestial: Bhagavad-Gita*. London: Routledge & Kegan Paul, Ltd., 1970. This famous and marvelous Sanskrit poem, translated from the Sanskrit by Sir Edwin Arnold, is a discourse between Arjuna, Prince of India and the Supreme Being in the form of Krishna.

Bahu, Dwight Condo. *T'ai Shan: An Account of the Sacred Eastern Peak of China*. Shanghai: The Commercial Press Ltd., 1925. This is an interesting account of the mountain T'ai Shan, its history and its importance.

Barnett, Michael C. *Transliterations of the Chinese Acupuncture Point Names with Explanations*. Occidental Institute Alumni Association, Summer Seminar/Workshop, 1982. Michael Barnett translated the information contained in this training material from the original French text titled *Traité d'Acuponcture Médicale, Tombe 1*, by Dr. Jean-Claude Darras.

Beijing College of Traditional Chinese Medicine. *Essentials of Chinese Acupuncture*. Beijing: Foreign Languages Press, 1980. This text is a very thorough treatment of the theory of acupuncture, complete with descriptions of the channels and their associated points. It also discusses the methods of treatment using acupuncture and moxibustion for many common ailments.

Chan, Wing-Tsit. *A Source Book in Chinese Philosophy*. Princeton: Princeton University Press, 1963. As the title suggests, this is a sourcebook of Chinese history and thought. It is invaluable to the Western student of Chinese philosophy.

Chatterji, J. C. *The Wisdom of the Vedas*. Wheaton, IL: Theosophical Publishing House, 1973. This exposition of India's outlook on life, based ultimately on the Vedas, explores how the most ancient wisdom of India regards life, its origin, purpose, and goals. A relatively short book, it is a well-written, concise work of deep scope.

Chen, Jing. *Anatomical Atlas of Chinese Acupuncture Points*. trans. Jiang, Qiyang, *et al*. Beijing: Shandong Science and Technology Press, 1980. This text is a very complete record, created especially for researchers who combine Traditional Chinese Medicine and acupuncture techniques with Western medicine. Since Qi Gong practitioners do not necessarily have medical training, the text serves this group best by indicating the specific acupuncture points and pathways of the channels. Such information is, of course, of critical importance to our discipline.

Chia, Mantak. *Awaken Healing Energy Through the Tao*. Santa Fe, NM: Aurora Press, 1983. The author presents a Taoist approach to the cultivation of the life energy, or chi, through descriptive analysis.

Conze, Edward. *Buddhist Scriptures*. London: Penguin Books, 1975. A collection of Buddhist writings compiled by an expert in Buddhism, this work was first translated in 1959, and it is a well–respected text.

Cook, Theodore Andrea. *The Curves of Life*. New York: Dover Publications, 1979. In the words of the subtitle, this profusely illustrated text, first published in 1914, is "An Account of the Spiral Formations and Their Application to Growth in Nature, to Science and to Art; with Special Reference to the Manuscripts of Leonardo da Vinci."

de Kleen, Tyra. *Mudras: The Ritual Hand–Poses of the Buddhist Priests and the Shiva Priests of Bali*. London: Kegan Paul, Trench, Turnbull & Co. Ltd., 1924. This work is an interesting and useful description of the history and purpose of the hand gestures the author found during her travels in Bali. The author has also sketched many of the mudras and noted their purpose.

Deussen, Pau. *The Philosophy of the Upanishads*. New York: Dover Publications, 1966. A philosophical treatise describing one of the most ancient of Eastern texts, *The Upanishads*, this text is not light reading, and is intended for the serious student of Eastern philosophy.

Esdaile, James. *Hypnosis in Medicine and Surgery*. New York: Julian Press, 1957. Dr. Esdaile presents a very factual (and fascinating) account of his experiences using Mesmerism (not hypnosis) in the treatment of clinically ill patients in India during the middle of the last century. It is well worth reading for those interested in the finer distinctions between the psychological techniques of hypnosis and the physical techniques relying on the use of Qi (prana.)

Govinda, Lama Anagarika. *The Way of the White Clouds*. Bombay: B.I. Publications, 1991. The Lama takes his readers on an unforgettable and spellbinding visit to Tibet before the Chinese occupation. He also explains many Tibetan mysteries in some detail.

Hartland, John. *Medical & Dental Hypnosis & Its Clinical Applications*. London: Baillière Tindall, 1982. This is an excellent sourcebook for anyone interested in the applications and techniques of hypnosis. It offers lengthy descriptions of scripts used in trance induction, methods to deepen the trance, and discusses the uses of hypnosis in specific clinical situations.

Jwing-Ming, Yang. *The Root of Chinese Chi Kung: The Secrets of Chi Kung Training*. Jamaica Plain, MA: Yang's Martial Arts Association (YMAA), 1989. This textbook contains the history and development of Chi Kung (Qi Gong), including its uses and theory.

Kaltenmark, Max. *Lao Tzu and Taoism*. Stanford, CA: Stanford University Press, 1969. This book describes the philosophy and life of Lao Tzu and includes a brief treatment of religious Taoism.

Kaptchuk, Ted J. *The Web That Has No Weaver*. New York: Congdon & Weed, 1983. Offering a detailed description of many aspects of Traditional Chinese Medicine, this book is an excellent place to begin reading in this vast field. It is also a reference text.

Krishna, Gopi. *Kundalini: the Evolutionary Energy in Man.* Boston: Shambhala, 1967. An autobiographical account of an extraordinary man's own experience with the awakening of Kundalini.

———. *Living With Kundalini.* Boston: Shambhala, 1993. This book is an expansion of his earlier work, *Kundalini: the Evolutionary Energy in Man,* and includes more personal autobiographical information than the original publication.

———. *The Wonder of the Brain.* Ontario: The F.I.N.D. Research Trust, 1987. This is a book that addresses the effects of prana, or life energy, on the brain and nervous system, written by the leading authority on Kundalini in this century.

Lade, Arnie. *Acupuncture Points: Images & Functions.* Seattle: Eastland Press, 1989. Restricting the scope of inquiry to about 250 acupuncture points, the author describes each anatomical location, the metaphoric image each name evokes and the traditional functions.

Latourette, Kenneth Scott. *The Chinese: Their History and Culture.* New York: Macmillan, 1934. A textbook on China, this reference work covers history, geography, and politics, but less philosophy than other books in this bibliography.

Liberman, Jacob. *Light: The Medicine of the Future.* Santa Fe, NM: Bear & Company, 1991. This text presents an interesting and relevant discussion of the effects of light and light therapy on our health and well-being.

Mitchell, Stephen. *Tao Te Ching.* New York: Harper Perennial, 1991. This is a recent English version of the *Tao Te Ching* and is translated with the contemporary Western reader in mind.

Mote, Frederick W. *Intellectual Foundations of China.* New York: Alfred A. Knopf, 1971. This is an historical account of China and its various philosophical movements.

Nicoll, Maurice. *The Mark.* London: Robinson and Watkins, 1954. A philosophical exposition for those seeking a greater understanding of the Christ teachings.

Pine, Red. *The Zen Teaching of Bodhidharma*. Berkeley, CA: North Point Press, 1987. *This is a translation of the teachings of the patriarch of Zen Buddhism, Bhodhidharma.*

Prabhavananda, Swami, and Frederick Manchester. *The Upanishads: Breath of the Eternal*. The Vedanta Society of Southern California. New York: Signet, 1975. This is an excellent translation of the oldest scriptures of India, *The Vedas*. All orthodox Hindus recognize these works as the origin of their faith and see them as their highest written authority.

Radha, Swami Sivananda. *The Divine Light Invocation*. British Columbia: Shiva Press, 1966. This small book contains historical information about Swami Radha's experience which culminated with the Divine Light Invocation and the actual practice of the Divine Light Mantra.

Radice, Betty, ed. *The Upanishads*. London: Penguin, 1965. *The Upanishads* are spiritual treatises of different lengths, the oldest of which were composed between 800 and 400 B.C. This is a collection of translations of some of the most famous.

Ramacharaka, Yogi. *The Bhagavad Gita, or the Message of the Master*. Chicago: Yogi Publication Society, 1930. A compilation from the best of the various good translations of this famous Hindu "Message of the Master."

_____. *Mystic Christianity: The Inner Teachings of the Master*. The Yogi Publication Society, Chicago, Illinois, 1907. This collection of lessons regarding the esoteric messages of the New Testament originally appeared in monthly form between October 1907 and November 1908. Each "chapter is in itself a lesson and meant to be studied in such a manner."

_____. *The Hindu-Yogi Science of Breath*. London: L.N. Fowler & Co., Ltd., 1960. The physical, psychic, mental, and spiritual aspects of the Yogic science of breath are discussed. The text is also an extensive reference source of exercises which are useful to athletes, singers, and those interested in promoting health, strength, and clarity of mind.

Shibayama, Abbot Zenkei. *A Flower Does Not Talk: Zen Essays*. Tokyo & Boston: Charles E. Tuttle, 1970. This collection of

Zen essays is prepared particularly for English-speaking people of the West by the abbot of the Nanzenji Monastery in Kyoto, Japan.

Snellgrove, David L., ed. *The Image of the Buddha*. Paris: Kodansha International (UNESCO), 1978. This work offers an outstanding collection of photographs specifically depicting the Buddha. The text sheds a great deal of light on the iconographic features of the images.

Suzuki, Daisetz Teitaro. *Studies in the Lankavatara Sutra*. Boston: Routledge & Kegan Paul, 1930. As one of the most important texts of Mahayana Buddhism, almost all of its principal tenets are presented, including the teaching of Zen.

Suzuki, Shunrya. *Zen Mind, Beginner's Mind*. New York: Weatherhill, 1970. This text, an introduction to the Zen way of thought, offers a practical approach to experiencing this in your daily life.

Teeguarden, Iona Marsaa. *Acupressure Way of Health: Jin Shin Do*. Tokyo & New York: Japan Publications, 1978. This is a practical guide to the acupressure technique known as Jin Shin Do. It contains many diagrams and useful, easy-to-read techniques and descriptions.

Wilhelm, Richard, trans. *The Secret of the Golden Flower*. London: Routledge & Kegan Paul, 1962. This translation of the *Chinese Book of Life* has both a foreword and commentary written by C. G. Jung. Wilhelm's book was first translated into English from the original German in 1931. It is a classic.

Xie, Zhufan. *Essentials of Traditional Chinese Medicine*. Hong Kong: The Commercial Press Ltd., 1984. Compiled by the Beijing Medical College, this text is a listing and description of the most common terms in Traditional Chinese Medicine in use today.

Index

H

I

J

K

About the Author

PETER FENTON HAS A PH.D. in Educational
Policy and Administrative Studies from the
University of Calgary, and has had a life-long
interest in nature and education. His background in philosophy, educational foundations and management theory, developing
curricula, the philosophy of science, the
heuristics of discovery, systems theory, tech-
nical training, the Internet, and an avid interest in the natural sciences, all combine to make
him an ideal teacher for Westerners who want
to become self-sufficient. He lives in Idaho,
where, with his wife, he has built his own
house.